Listening to in Psychotherapy

CH00920266

Mary Butterton

Senior Accredited Practitioner,
British Association for Counselling and Psychotherapy
Graduate of the Royal Scottish Academy of Music and Drama

Foreword by

Colwyn Trevarthen

Radcliffe Publishing

Oxford • New York

Radcliffe Publishing Ltd
18 Marcham Road
Abingdon
Oxon OX14 1AA
United Kingdom

www.radcliffe-oxford.com
Electronic catalogue and worldwide online ordering facility.

© 2008 Mary Butterton

All rights reserved. No part of this publication may be reproduced, stored in a retrieval system or transmitted, in any form or by any means, electronic, mechanical, photocopying, recording or otherwise without the prior permission of the copyright owner.

Mary Butterton has asserted her right under the Copyright, Designs and Patents Act, 1998, to be identified as Author of this Work.

Neither the publisher nor the authors accept liability for any injury or damage arising from this publication.

British Library Cataloguing in Publication Data

A catalogue record for this book is available from the British Library.

ISBN-13 978 1 85775 741 5

Typeset by Anne Joshua & Associates, Oxford
Printed and bound by TJI Digital, Padstow, Cornwall

Contents

Foreword

A new, more present, psychodynamics

When Mary Butterton invites a patient to bring 'special' music into the consulting room, the balance between being in the present and causes found in the past is changed, and so is the patient–therapist relationship. Mary's book is about, 'the meaning of music for the patient and psychotherapist. In particular for the psychotherapist who in the past has shied away from allowing music to be chosen and brought into the consulting room by the patient'. It involves a change of the meaning of 'meaning', making it more like 'being with, now'. It also brings the word 'dynamic' to life in what Daniel Stern calls 'the present moment in psychotherapy and everyday life'.[1] Time is changed.

For the Danish jazz musician and semiotician Ole Kühl it is clear. 'What we share in music is not just sound, but also, and perhaps more importantly, time. We share *structured time*, when we share music. When we hear music, we entrain to a pulse, while we synchronise ourselves cognitively to a temporal pattern of expectations and predictions, set up through musical form and gestures'.[2] Music is about the Self alive, about the time and tensions of moving. Its experience is free of the named facts of memory, and it can think or feel in new ways about the future – about who the person alive in the music is, what kind of person 'I am and will be', with what kind of hopes and anxieties, and about the people who are 'my friends'. Its meanings are implicit and need no explication. It moves with miraculous ease between us, in both imagination and memory. It becomes a cultural 'habitus' we accept to live within.

The four notable people Mary interviews here about their love of music find it in different places: 'out there' in the appreciated world, within their Self, or in relationships alive between people. Clearly music inhabits a world between the intimate, the private, the public, the ordinary and the very 'special'. It lives as in the·innocent creations of 'children's musical culture' observed by the Norwegian musicologist Jon-Roar Bjørkvold, with their surprising premonitions of high musical art.[3] But in the end, there are immutable 'values' that all music must preserve, inseparable from human moods, profound and lasting or superficial and transitory as these may be. In its wordless power the mimesis of music is one manifestation of a mind that needs culture.

Mary's absorbing overview of philosophical, sociological, psychological, and neuroscientific theories of what music is, clears the way for deep appreciation of music therapy and especially for understanding how listening to and sharing of special music may engage the client's Self and that of the therapist, how it may engage a patient whose recollections of distress lead to a wordless isolation – 'in this prototypic state, this place before words, the client may come alive to the sound of emotionally significant music'. We are told how one woman's chosen music opened the way to a musical companionship with her therapist that allowed her to retrieve experiences of being a loved and happy child. Liz moved, from immobility in a sad story built of words and fragmented memories of childhood hurts, into the present life of her body, between its pain and capacity for pleasure. She was able to step away from severe psychosomatic distress or hold it at a distance, so the pleasure or 'flow' of being could be shared.

All of us who have observed closely the making of dialogues of meaning between infants and affectionate adults are impressed by its rhythmic efficiency and emotional fluency – by its 'musicality' and 'companionship'. We also observe the immediate withdrawal and sadness when the infant's hopes for company are disappointed. This meeting of minds through body movement is the 'cradle of thought' that Peter Hobson writes about, which nurtures the earliest meaning making between the child and others.[4] Its emotions of intersubjective 'attunement', and the 'dynamic emotional envelopes', as Daniel Stern describes them, are strong and can be both creative and destructive.[5] They can change the way the infant's brain grows. The genius for making human sense, its innate intersubjectivity, is not implanted in the infant by adult wisdom. As the happy parent knows, the baby is an intuitive maker and learner of meanings. Meaningful encounters with him or her are soon full of imaginative invention and the making of memorable rituals.

Advances in brain science bring new understanding, allowing recognition of the influence on cognition of vital intuitions and emotions of moving and communicating that had been neglected or denied. But neuroscience is often misled by accidental correlations of convenient measurement, by biases of evidence due to its intrinsic technical limitations, especially the relative ease with which single heads can be studied in artificial conditions where moving is severely limited, and by reductive assumptions about causes and effects in cognitive processes. Research on communicative musicality of infants underlines a need for a biochronology of the brain, for attention to the clocks of body and mind that regulate vital activities from moments to lifetimes, and especially for the brain functions that enable the times of life to be shared between persons.

We have inherited a theory of mind that gives an account of beliefs and desires as products of the reception, processing and retention of information by an impressionable mechanism, detached from the time of bodily experience – too dependent upon the arbitrary certainty of language. This theory is challenged by the impulsive drama of life, by the vitality of expression in dance and music and in the prosody and gestures of live speaking, which communicates the beliefs and desires of a person speaking to other persons, as well as any facts they may assert.

This is a book about a new more vital way of understanding the human spirit, and it offers a different way of managing a therapeutic relationship, one that invites the patient to gain hope and pleasure from the rhythm and sympathy of music.

Colwyn Trevarthen
September 2007

References

1 Stern DN (2004) *The Present Moment: in psychotherapy and everyday life*. Norton, New York.
2 Kühl O (2007) *Musical Semantics* (European Semiotics: Language, Cognition and Culture. No. 7). Peter Lang, Bern.
3 Bjørkvold J-R (1992) *The Muse Within: creativity and communication, song and play from childhood through maturity*. Harper Collins, New York.
4 Hobson P (2002) *The Cradle of Thought: exploring the origins of thinking*. Macmillan, London.
5 Stern DN (2000) *The Interpersonal World of the Infant: a view from psychoanalysis and development psychology*. Basic Books, New York.

Preface

This book was written because I needed to understand more of what might be happening in the psychotherapeutic process when music, chosen by the patient, was brought into the consulting room. Some patients, invited by me, brought music in when there did not seem to be any words available to them to communicate the intense feelings they were seen and felt to be experiencing. It seemed that these patients were those who had suffered the early trauma of loss and had no verbal memory of it.

I started to ask if there was music that they might want to listen to with me when these periods of silent emptiness began to appear more often in the session. I invited the patients to bring in CDs that were important to them. The shift and movement in the therapeutic process was encouraging. New verbal material was brought into the sessions and significant relational memories were talked about for the first time.

I was aware that listening to music which is important for the listener reached deeply into early memories[1] but I felt that more understanding of the process of the therapeutic effect of listening to music, shared with the therapist in the consulting room, was necessary. More needed to be understood about the experience of listening to music in general, and this began an enquiry into the philosophy, psychology, sociology and neuroscience of music and how persons experience it.

Neuroscience, however, and in particular the work of Trevarthen[2] and Malloch[3] seemed to be the place where music and the early inner mental life of persons came together. Their research work into the shared experience of musicality, which is called communicative musicality, between the infant and mother/carer, was very important in my enquiry. Their work included early shared experience of passages of music, that is, early baby songs. Here, at last, was a theory of musicality and music which was grounded in evidence-based research which I felt could be built on. It is hoped that this book will encourage research into the shared experience of music within psychotherapy.

Mary Butterton
September 2007

References

1 Butterton M (2004) *Music and Meaning: opening minds in the caring and healing professions*. Radcliffe Medical Press, Oxford.
2 Trevarthen C (1999) Musicality and the intrinsic motive pulse: evidence from human psycho-biology and infant communication. *Musicae Scientiae*. Special Issue 1999–2000. The European Society for Cognitive Sciences, Belgium, p. 155.
3 Malloch S (1999) Mothers and infants and communicative musicality. *Musicae Scientiae*. Special Issue 1999–2000. The European Society for Cognitive Sciences, Belgium, p. 48.

About the author

Mary Butterton is a graduate of the Royal Scottish Academy of Music and Drama and is a Senior Accredited Practitioner with the British Association for Counselling and Psychotherapy. She has taught and lectured on music appreciation for many years as well as teaching psychodynamic counselling and working as a music psychotherapist in the NHS. She is particularly interested in the personal experience of listening to music. She has a PhD in music, psychotherapy and theology from the University of Birmingham and now works in private practice in Derby.

Acknowledgements

Many people have made this book possible and I cannot claim that it was written by me alone. First, I would like to thank Mercedes Pavlicevic, Katie Melua, Baroness Neuberger and Benjamin Zephaniah for starting the book off with their personal experiences of listening to music. Their writings are deeply personal and truly generous accounts. It is Liz, however, I have to thank especially for her psychotherapeutic contribution. Her case material is the core of the book.

The work of many researchers informed my understanding and reflection on music and persons especially in neuroscience and the therapeutic process, and I am deeply indebted to them.

There are many people I wish to thank for their unfailing support in this new venture – Antonia Murphy and Fiona Aitken deserve special thanks for kindly contributing their casework material in the Coda; also Sue Phillips and John Neat for reading chapters of the script; and Margaret Wilkinson, Pat Bryant, Maggie Senior, Anne Shotter, Mandy Rolland-Smith and all at Radcliffe Publishing for their generous help and support.

Lastly, I want to thank my husband Harold, and two adult children, Alice and Andrew, for putting up with me having half a brain preoccupied with writing.

To my husband Harold, and Alice and Andrew

Introduction

This book is about the meaning of music for the patient and psychotherapist. In particular it is for the psychotherapist who in the past has shied away from allowing music to be chosen and brought into the consulting room by the patient.

The experience of listening to music has been explored through the related disciplines of sociology, psychology, anthropology and neuroscience and has been informed by writings in psychoanalytic psychotherapy, attachment theory and psychoanalysis. The aim of this book is to draw attention to the need for more research into music within psychotherapy with children and adults who have suffered early emotional trauma in childhood. We already know that just like all of us they can be reached through music where words seem to fail, but as yet we don't know enough about how and why this is so. In these pages there is an attempt to begin to articulate some answers.

This book concentrates on the receptive *listening* experience of music. As noted above, in listening to music within psychotherapy the music is *chosen by the patient*. This choice of music by the patient is central to this form of therapy. Also the music that the patient brings into the consulting room will be understood to be particularly important for them and as music that they *need* to listen to with another human being at that time.

The discipline of music therapy

Much research has been and is being done in traditional music therapy but what is being offered here is different from the active engagement with musical instruments that characterises what we generally understand music therapy to be. However, there *is* a form of *listening* to music within the established music therapy world. This is called Guided Imagery and Music (GIM). Here the music is usually chosen by the therapist and this again is very different from listening to music in psychotherapy as described in this book.

This raises the question 'Why has music within psychotherapy not been written about before?' It must be the case that the patient's interest in listening to music has come up in psychotherapy before now. But there may be at least

GIM: Music chosen by the therapist.

1

two reasons for this. The first is that this kind of musical therapeutic engagement may have been thought to be the province of GIM therapists.

Here there is extensive musical training involved in the method and on choosing programmes of music in consultation with the patient. It is therefore understandable that psychotherapists have not written about listening to music before. Another reason why listening to music in psychotherapy seems to have been neglected is that, as has been noted above, traditional music therapy has concentrated on active musical participation with a variety of musical instruments, which again requires long specialist training.

In the National Health Service listening to music with groups of patients has been tried in psychiatric hospital settings but problems arose around the choice of music. Music chosen by the therapist was felt not to be acceptable to the whole group.[1] Another point is that, as far as is known, the practice of listening to music within individual psychotherapy may well be going on but it has not been written up simply because not enough is known about how it works.

The new interdisciplinary thinking and research in affective neuroscience and music of Panksepp and Bekkedal[2] and in the psychology of music by Juslin and Sloboda[3] along with the cognitive neuroscience of music of Peretz and Zatorre,[4] and Trevarthen and Malloch's work on 'communicative musicality'[5] is beginning to change this lack of knowledge. What is needed now is some evidence-based research into psychotherapy with individual adults on the experience of listening to music within therapy. This book aims to raise awareness of the need for such research especially in work with adults who may have suffered trauma in early childhood before there were words to begin to talk about their inner pain.

Listening to music in the context of individual psychotherapy will be described in some detail in Chapter 10 'A two-part invention'. This is a description of psychotherapeutic sessions with Liz, in which listening to music chosen by her was an important feature. I try to illustrate, in this chapter, that music used as a therapeutic medium can access memories for the patient which have been previously inaccessible through words. It will then be reflected upon in the light of modern attachment theory and writings in psychology, sociology and neuroscience. Aspects of the clinical therapeutic work done by two other psychotherapists will be presented in Chapter 14 to remind us that music *does* come into the consulting room.

What is so special about listening to music within psychotherapy?

In this book the shared experience of listening to music, followed by the patient's descriptions of the experience of listening to music, may be seen to assist the process of psychotherapy, especially when this process reaches an impasse and words are no longer available to the patient. In these circumstances music is a medium and a means of right-brain-to-right-brain communication to the therapist; what the patient needs to have the therapist know and feel. It would seem that aspects of some patients' inner states are held in their choice of music. In the conversation following this shared experience, the patient will usually attempt to verbalise or 'say more' about the shared experience and this may be communicated in part by gesture, the liveliness (or not) of the body, in other words through their 'communicative musicality', to borrow a phrase from Stephen Malloch.[6] They may even feel that they want to paint or write an account of their experience as Liz has done in this book. That would really be bringing their inner experience into words!

All of this will take some time but Schore writes that the therapist should hold this right-brain-to-right-brain felt experience until it has been 'lived with' for some time in the consulting room.[7] Listening to music affords this kind of 'lived time' for both the patient and the therapist.

In listening to music within psychodynamic psychotherapy we try to understand something of the inner dynamics of what is going on in the patient's mind, and how they relate to the therapist. What their choice of music means for them is then explored in the room. First, however, we need to map out the terrain of music and the terrain of persons. This will give us a language with which to underpin this enquiry.

Dynamic fields

It is known that there are several dynamic fields operating in psychodynamic word-based psychotherapy itself. There is the dynamic field of persons-in-relationship within the patient's mind, that is, their inner world is populated with memories and feelings from their past and present life. There is then the dynamic field of the inner individual private self-in-relationship world of the therapist outside the room, which should be attended to and then put to one side, as it were. There is then the complex dynamic field of the relationship between patient and therapist with transference, counter-transference and the working alliance relationship (which will be explained more fully in Chapter 11).

This is nothing new here and psychodynamic psychotherapists work within these dynamic fields every day. However, listening to music within psychotherapy adds the overlapping dynamic field of the motion of tones that make up the passages and patterns of sound in the chosen music. How the felt meaning of these chosen passages of music is understood by the patient, what it symbolises for them, as it overlaps with the felt meaning of their past interpersonal experiences must be heard, felt and understood in communication with the therapist. Furthermore, how all of this is held in the relationship to the therapist is the stuff of this book.

But where are these dynamic fields?

When reference is made to 'dynamic fields' in this book we are talking about connecting patterns of neurones in the brain. These connecting patterns would have arisen in infancy in relationship with the mother and/or our first carers. This would have been right-brain-to-right-brain communication between infant and carer, before the more mature connections with the left brain are formed and verbal language comes on stream between ages 2–3 years. Schore writes that 'The maternal comforting strata resides in the mother's right brain, the hemisphere that is dominant for non-verbal behaviour and for responding to stress.'[7]

Although adults do not have verbal access to this early period of self-in-relationship, there are traces in every infant's brain that may be reached in adult psychotherapy through right-brain-to-right-brain methods of engagement. Listening to music chosen by the patient engages in just this kind of right-brain-to-right-brain therapeutic and comforting activity. This may enable later dis-regulated ways of being-in-relationship to emerge in the consulting room and be worked through in the relationship with the therapist who has shared this early right-brain way of being-in-relationship. Listening to music chosen by the patient in psychotherapy may access these early relational patterns quite directly as the musical patterns and shapes chosen by the patient may overlap with traces of their felt right-brain experiences of a nurturing mother or carer. This early experience may pre-date any trauma of loss that the patient may have experienced and the therapist's task would be to model a more benign later-developing process for the patient. Because music may reach these early right-brain experiences more directly, the length of time within psychotherapy may be reduced. It is suggested here that the early heard and felt patterns of nurture to be found in traces in the patient's brain which resonate through listening to their music will hopefully be mirrored by the therapist. The repetition of this right-brain-to-right-brain process may then begin to re-build a new more secure base of self-in-relationship for the patient. This right-brain-to-right-brain repetition within psychotherapy is advocated by Schore when working with early relational trauma.[7] He writes:

> 'It is important to again stress that early relational trauma, attachment psychopathology, and the defences of dissociation are stored in the right hemisphere. The emergence of strong affect during psychotherapy sessions is known to be accompanied by increased right-hemispheric activation in the patient. And thus in these central moments of the treatment of developmentally disordered patients, holding the right-brain-to-right-brain context of emotional communication is essential.'

The bigger picture

Although the experience of listening to music within psychotherapy is concerned with the individual person-in-relationship rather than a social grouping, this bigger social perspective has informed the writing in this book more fully about the experience of listening to music in the one-to-one relationship in the consulting room. This is because, as Sloboda writes, the individual person is completely enmeshed in a social and cultural world.[8] It is the patient's *choice* of music that is important in psychotherapy and we do need to understand as much as possible about the cultural context and beginnings of any patient's musical experience.

Much work has been done on the experience of listening to music with groups of people within different cultures. This knowledge will inform our receptive position to the patient's chosen music in the consulting room. For example, the patient's cultural life may be embedded in the experience of 'rock music' and the therapist's understanding of this aspect of the patient's culture will be necessary in order for empathic resonance to occur between them, that is, right-brain-to-right-brain communication.

In this book what this kind of musical experience might mean for an individual person will be further understood and better informed within the context of psychotherapy by approaching other disciplines and enquiring how the *experience* of listening to music is understood from that particular perspective. Some of the findings from the philosophy of music, from evolutionary psychology, sociology, affective neuroscience, attachment theory and musicology will assist in a broader understanding of what it is, in the patient's musical encounter, that holds real importance for them as these disciplines touch on the special experience of listening to music in the consulting room.

Part 1

To begin the exploration of what is really the personal aesthetic experience of an individual listening to music within psychotherapy, we will start outside the context of psychotherapy. Four people in the public eye have kindly agreed to talk about what music means for each of them

In Chapters 1–4 Mercedes Pavlicevic, Katie Melua, Baroness Neuberger and Benjamin Zephaniah have each kindly agreed to be interviewed about their experience of music and what it means for them. They agreed to this very personal type of interview because they are all sympathetic to the need for more research into how music can help the healing of early trauma in the young and old. In the conversations on what music means for them they allow us to glimpse something of the truth of who they are as persons-in-relationship. Because music is able to reach very deeply into our emotional experiences I am greatly indebted to each of them for agreeing to reveal so much of their inner world.

In Chapter 5, we try to sum up what we understand and now know about the musical experiences of the four interviewees.

Part 2

In Part 2 we turn to music itself. In order to take some care to broaden and deepen our understanding of the experience of music, we turn to other disciplines that consider music from their own particular perspectives.

Chapter 6 begins with the very basic question, 'What exactly is music?' Here we call upon the philosophy of music for assistance. However, this would seem to be a daunting task because there is much disagreement between philosophers themselves on exactly what music is and how we are said to experience it.[9,10] This is interesting as it emphasises that we all perceive music slightly differently. We might disagree with our neighbour on how it is perceived but so do the philosophers!! We turn to Zuckerkandl's thinking on music as motion in the dynamic field of tones and then link this with Langer's ideas of music as a symbol of the structure of our emotional life, to try to move nearer to understanding something about the human experience of listening to music.[11,12] We also touch on Cumming's thinking on music as in relation to persons.[13] This attempts to link the listener's outer and inner experience of music.

Then we look to the sociologists for help in the hope that the study of groups of *persons* and music might throw some light on the nature of musical experience.

Chapter 7 approaches the psychology of the experience of music. Here we find an exploration of 'everyday music' and 'special music'. We consider social psychology where Sloboda and O'Neill[14] and De Nora[15] have studied 'everyday music' as self-therapy, but Sloboda and O'Neill themselves observe that this personal manipulation of emotions by an individual person practising self-therapy is not the same as the therapy that helps an individual to manage life's difficulties.[16]

In Chapter 8 attention is drawn to the contextual aspect or 'habitus' of the experience of listening to music. This has special relevance for the practice of listening to music within psychotherapy because psychotherapy is a very particular relational context. It is also noted in this chapter that brain study research on the experience of music has traditionally been the study of single brains.

Becker's thinking from an anthropological perspective draws our attention to the 'habitus' of the experience of music.[17] This 'habitus' of listening to music necessarily involves the other person. The contribution of current musicology is then noted in the writing and experiential work of some modern musicologists. Here there is a movement towards descriptions of the experience of music from a Jungian perspective and a new interest linking the experience of persons and music is detected.

Before describing in outline the practice of listening to music within psychotherapy, we consider traditional active Music Therapy alongside Guided

Imagery and Music, which is the listening experience within the traditional discipline of Music Therapy. This branch of Music Therapy is one in which the *therapist chooses* a prescribed programme of listening to music with the patient. We consider both Christoph Schwabe's 'Resource-Oriented Music Therapy' and Isabelle Frohne-Hagemann's 'Artistic Media and Music Therapy' as being particularly bound up with personal relations.[18,19] Lars Ole Bonde's work is of particular interest because of his current research into the Bonny Method of Guided Imagery in Music (BMGIM) in the rehabilitation of cancer patients.[20]

The experiential core of music and persons is reached in Chapter 9. Here the *origin* of the adult self-in-relationship in neuroscience and music is considered. The work of Stephen Malloch and Colwyn Trevarthen on infant/mother communicative musicality is presented as underpinning the practice of listening to music within psychotherapy.[6,21] Here we are reminded that we must start at our beginnings. We have all been babies at one time, maybe in the far distant past, but our brains began to be sculpted in those first early engagements with our carers, especially the mother or other primary carer. These basic sub-cortical brain structures and the later patterns of neurones which fire in the adult processes of thinking and feeling have their origins in this early well-spring of who we were as growing infants in attachment to our mother or first carer(s).

Because our earliest experiences of music arise from our earliest relationships, Chapter 9 describes in outline the 'good enough' infant–mother dynamic engagement and discusses the dynamic feeling content of such a relationship. In this book these earliest dynamic patterns in the brain, musical and affective, will be said to resonate with dynamic patterns in music that is of deep personal importance for us, especially in therapy.

In this chapter the deep structures in music, tonal and rhythmic, and the deep structures in our early developing right-brain attachment with mother will be seen to come together in the work of Trevarthen on infant–mother communicative musicality.[22] It is the author's hypothesis that, through listening to music chosen by the patient within psychotherapy, the experience of these traces of an early patterning of 'good enough' self-in-relationship will be matched in the musical patterning chosen by the patient. This early musical patterning may again be engaged with through music chosen by the patient in a trusted interpersonal relationship. When memories behind the trauma begin to come to words, new neural pathways are made available for the patient. How this is further worked through developmentally in further sessions is the stuff of this particular form of music in psychotherapy.

Part 3

Chapter 10 is called a 'Two-part invention' and is a description of a single case study of Liz. In the world of music a 'two-part invention' is understood to refer to a famous book of contrapuntal writing for the keyboard by JS Bach. Two-part contrapuntal writing means that two lines of music, or two 'voices' imitate one another and weave around one another in interesting ways but always making room for each other. There are many contrapuntal devices used in two-part inventions, for example, one voice or chosen melodic phrase may use notes of longer time value while the other voice plays the first presented version of note values. This is known as augmentation. The opposite device of diminution might also be used. This would be to write the notes of the chosen melodic phrase in shorter time values, which would be played against the first presented version of the chosen melodic phrase. Another device might be 'stretto', which is an overlapping of the two parts or voices, or the two parts both being played at a quicker tempo.

This chapter is a description of clinical case material with Liz when she began to bring music she wanted to listen to into the consulting room. She very kindly agreed to some of our work together being included in this book and she herself contributed much of the written material in Chapter 10 and the reader may find, within the writing, examples of the musical contrapuntal devices of augmentation, diminution and stretto in verbal form.

Liz had worked in verbal psychotherapy with me for several years but after we had finished she had a bad experience while attending a pain clinic. She chose to re-enter therapy with me in June 2003 and agreed that we work together using listening to music which was important for her. The account of this casework dates from June 2003 until July 2004.

In Chapter 11 the case material is reflected upon and psychological understanding of the dynamic relational work is presented.

Chapter 12 analyses the musical choices Liz made in the context of enhanced communicative musicality. A symbolic developmental narrative will be seen to emerge in Liz's musical choices as she works through her grief and sorrow and finds her mature voice-in-relationship in her creative writing.

Chapter 13 asks the question 'Where are we now?' The journey from exploring the experience of listening to music with our four interviewees through finding more about what music means in terms of philosophy, psychology and neuroscience is reviewed along with the case study. An attempt will be made to show how important communicative musicality is and how it links music and persons in the experience of listening to music within the consulting room. In this attempt at integration it is hoped that the reader will recognise more of what music might mean in their own life and how it is a medium that could be used to facilitate the recovery from early traumatic states of being-in-relationship. It is hoped that future research may be developed in this area.

The book ends with a coda in Chapter 14. This again is a musical term and not one usually used to describe a chapter in a book, but as this book is about the overlap of the experience of words and music in the consulting room I shall be creative! In the *Oxford Dictionary of Music* a coda is said to be a movement at the end of music to clinch matters or to have an integral formal significance.[23] In this book the coda does not *clinch* matters but it *does* have a formal significance. It describes some of the work of two psychotherapists, Antonia

Murphy and Fiona Aitken, and what happened for them in their practice when music came into their consulting room. Although it doesn't clinch matters, this coda opens the field to further discussion and it does have formal significance in that it underlines the need for early agreement between therapist and patient that music be brought into the consulting room by the patient.

References

1 Wigram T (1995) *The Art and Science of Music Therapy: A handbook.* Harwood Academic Publishers, Newark NJ.
2 Panksepp J and Bekkedal M (1997) The affective cerebral consequences of music. *International Journal of Arts-Medicine.* **5:** 18–27.
3 Juslin P and Sloboda J (eds) (2001) *Music and Emotion.* Oxford University Press, Oxford.
4 Peretz I and Zatorre R (eds) (2003) *The Cognitive Neuroscience of Music.* Oxford University Press, Oxford.
5 Trevarthen C and Malloch S (2002) The musical lives of babies and families. *Journal of Zero to Three: National Center for Infants, Toddlers and Families.* 23(1): 11.
6 Malloch S (1999) Mothers and infants and communicative musicality. *Musicae Scientiae.* Special Issue (1999–2000). The European Society for Cognitive Sciences, Belgium, pp. 29–57.
7 Schore A (2003) *Affect Regulation.* WW Norton & Company, London, p. 94.
8 Juslin P and Sloboda J (eds) (2001) *Music and Emotion.* Oxford University Press, Oxford, p. 428.
9 Budd M (1985) *Music and the Emotions.* Routledge and Kegan Paul, London.
10 Scruton R (1999) *The Aesthetics of Music.* Oxford University Press, Oxford.
11 Zuckerkandl V (1956) *Sound and Symbol.* Bollingen Series XLIV. Princeton University Press, Princeton NJ.
12 Langer S (1942) *Philosophy in a New Key.* Harvard University Press, Cambridge, Mass.
13 Cumming N (2000) *The Sonic Self.* Indiana University Press, Bloomington, Indianapolis.
14 Sloboda J and O'Neill S (2001) Emotion in everyday listening to music. In: P Juslin and J Sloboda (eds) *Music and Emotion.* Oxford University Press, Oxford, p. 415.
15 De Nora T (2001) Aesthetic agency and musical practice: new directions in the sociology of music and emotion. In: P Juslin and J Sloboda (eds) *Music and Emotion.* Oxford University Press, Oxford, p. 169.
16 Sloboda J and O'Neill S (2001) Emotions in everyday listening to music. In: P Juslin and J Sloboda (eds) *Music and Emotion.* Oxford University Press, Oxford, p. 426.
17 Becker J (2004) *Deep Listeners.* Indiana University Press. Bloomington, Indianapolis.
18 Schwabe C (2005) Resource-orientated music therapy. *Nordic Journal of Music Therapy.* **14**(1): 53.
19 Frohne-Hagemann I (2005) Artistic media and music therapy. *Nordic Journal of Music Therapy.* **14**(2): 165–7.
20 Bonde LO (2005) Finding a new place. Metaphor and narrative in one cancer survivor's BMGIM therapy. *Nordic Journal of Music Therapy.* **14**(2): 137–54.
21 Trevarthen C (1999) Musicality and the intrinsic motive pulse: evidence from

human psychobiology and infant communication. *Musicae Scientiae.* Special Issue (1999–2000). The European Society for Cognitive Sciences, Belgium, pp. 155–211.

22 Trevarthen C (2002) Intrinsic motives for companionship in understanding: their origin, development and significance for infant mental health. *Infant Mental Health Journal.* **22**(1–2): 95–131.

23 Kennedy M (ed.) (1994) *The Oxford Dictionary of Music* (2e). Oxford University Press, Oxford.

PART 1

Experiencing Music

CHAPTER 1

Conversation with Mercedes Pavlicevic

Mercedes Pavlicevic is a Professor of Music Therapy in South Africa.

I live in Africa where driving is generally a more spacious business than in Europe. My best listening time is when I drive. I have a CD wallet with about 39 CDs, which I update regularly depending on what I have bought recently, or what I haven't listened to for a long time. On my way to and from work (20–30 minutes each way), this is my private quiet space and my car has a good sound system, so I 'chill'. My choice depends a lot on my mood – and within seconds I know whether or not I feel like this or that piece of music, and change immediately. When it is the 'wrong' music, I can't bear it, and if unable to change CDs (because I'm driving), then I switch off rather than listen to the wrong music. Listening takes my mind off the traffic and the day (especially after work) and helps me to 'flow'. Music also makes my car a special place – my space for ME – and whenever someone else gets in the car the first thing I do is switch off the CD player. So I love my car because of this (no I don't especially like driving – it is more about this delicious privacy, which is a rich time of the day for me). After my yoga class (twice a week) I cannot listen to music at all. I drive in silence.

Home is not an especially good place for listening, mainly because my partner is a musician and we have different musical tastes. Also we're both sensitive to what is being played and how and I have a feeling that she tends to listen when I'm not at home.

The kind of music I like is – difficult to say – except that it needs to be 'expressive', not just chuntering along. I say this because someone recently gave me a CD of the Orchestre de Baobab. They play African genre – wonderful orchestration and good melodies – but somehow it doesn't work for me; there's something mechanical about it and I get bored. So I need music that breathes, and enables me to breathe too, in a flowing way. I have a wonderful CD by Inti-Illimani, which is a Chilean group. They play mainly acoustic instruments, and they are BRILLIANT musicians; very sensitive, expressive and utterly deli-cious. Yo Yo Ma is another artist I love, because of this exquisite ultra-sensitivity and virtuosity. That's it – it is virtuosity that I love in music. Not a show-off kind of virtuosity, but being utterly accomplished and above that, music so it just plays itself or plays you (as we music therapists like to say). And when I listen to artists like this then the music and I become one; I lose sense of the day, or time or place and become this energy that flows me, in a way, and allows me to allow it to flow me (if that makes sense). I think it has more to do with my body than my mind – I listen and become it with my entire being, not just my mind. Hence my going on about breathing.

I have a wide range of tastes. In the classics I listen to a lot of Bach; adore Brahms – the colour of his music is magical; and Prokofiev too, and Shostako-vich. Then I listen to a lot of African music, Youssou N'dour, Ismael Lo – brilliant Senegalese musicians who sing in a mixture of English, French Arabic, and their own language – and music from the Portuguese African colonies is also wonderful. Then stuff from Sting, Simon and Garfunkel, Abba sometimes. Then there are the Beatles, Eric Clapton, kd lang, some African Gospel is wonderful, Anne Murray, Ella Fitzgerald (gorgeous musician) . . . Nusrat Ali Khan . . . Much of it music from my teens and twenties.

And I adore opera. When in London I inevitably will go. I like to go alone and become absorbed in it without needing to talk about it – which often interrupts the experience. And music is also linked to my Roman Catholic upbringing. I grew up in Rome, in the time of the Latin rite, and we attended Mass at the Vatican with lots of singing . . . and I love the spectacle of music and worship, which is an essential part of my culture even though I don't practise.

Almost inevitably I have a tune in my head – it seems to go on without necessarily my being aware of it. But if I stop and think I can tell you what it is. (It is a Bach prelude at the minute.)

MB: Mercedes, you write that your choice of music depends on your mood and it seems that music helps your mood and I'm wondering what might be going on here? Could you say a bit more about this? Does music help you check how you are feeling? Or is it something different?

Mercedes: I don't think that music helps me identify my mood – it's almost the other way round in that it is often my mood that helps me to choose the music I listen to and I will choose music that reflects my mood, or amplifies it, or that maybe shifts it. So, most of the time, if I am going to listen to music, the music of my choice that's different from the radio . . . There's a very quick check as to what I feel like and what's going on around me. I think you can translate it into what mood I'm in and what musical mood I'm in, in relation to what music I'm going to listen to . . . if that makes sense . . . (shared laughter). If I feel like remaining in the same mood I will choose one piece of music, but if I feel like having my mood shifted or amplified I may well choose something different.

MB: Yes . . . Could you give me an example?

Mercedes: I might think I feel like something Latin American and I put it on and then think 'Oh no . . . that doesn't feel quite right, doesn't quite fit somehow.'

MB: Right.

Mercedes: If it fits I won't think about it, I'll just know.

MB: Yes . . . so it's almost as if there is a second check . . . not a very conscious check when you start but then the second check moves in and you re-arrange your choice, if you like?

Mercedes: Yes, exactly.

MB: Would it be that music is a baseline truth that you tap into?

Mercedes: I think of it as more like a beacon or as a harbour or an anchor. It is something that . . . allows safety . . . the familiarity of it and the varying distance . . . sometimes you can feel very close to a beacon and other times very far away. I have been listening to the Beatles recently. I found a collection. When I was young the Beatles were making the headlines . . . I was pre-teens, so I was aware that this music was going on . . . and when I listen to it now (and I listen to it as a musician), I think what brilliant music. Listen to what they managed to do. And other times I listen and think . . . oh tinny sound . . . poor technology . . . I can really hear we're 40 years further on. I think I also listen in different ways so that's why the baseline of truth doesn't quite fit my truth as a musician, my truth as a person, my truth as an emoting being, my truth as a researcher, etc.

MB: And you need to check all of these when you say 'truth'?

Mercedes: Yes, absolutely.

MB: When you write that music helps you to flow, can you say something more here? Where is this flow? Can you situate it? Does it belong to the physical body or does it include the psyche . . .?

Mercedes: I think it's more of a sensate flow. I don't distinguish between the psyche and my body and the senses . . . I think they are absolutely integrated.

MB: Yes.

Mercedes: Mmn . . . so that when I think of flow I think of it literally as kinaesthetic.

MB: Movement.

Mercedes: Movement and feeling and touch and pressure and intensity and weight . . . all of these things.

MB: It is now generally accepted that as a baby develops in the womb, movement and sound are very much its experience at this early time.

Mercedes: And temperature and warmth.

MB: And Stephen Cross writes that babies are primed for music in the womb. This would also be Trevarthen's thinking too, wouldn't it?

Mercedes: Yes, in terms of basic capacity for it. Mmn . . .

MB: But I think that you are saying that all of you is immersed in the experience of music?

Mercedes: I think though there are times when certain kinds of music don't make sense. And that's a cognitive thing . . . like when I first heard Pierrot Lunaire. It was at the Usher Hall in Edinburgh and it was a brilliant perform-ance, or so people said. I think it was *Amsterdam Concertgebouw* – Bernard Haitink.

MB: Yes.

Mercedes: And I felt completely outside this music . . . I could not make sense of it.

MB: Yes, that's difficult when that happens isn't it?

Mercedes: But my musicianship was activated because I was trying to decode it . . . make sense of it . . . and I couldn't. I wouldn't say I was repelled by it but I was a bit puzzled. Couldn't make sense of it at all. I remained outside it.

MB: Yes that's an interesting thought . . . to remain outside of some experience like that.

Mercedes: And it was very curious because it was in a public domain. So it was a live musicking and the audience was enraptured and I thought 'What *is* this? I can't make sense of this music'.

MB: This brings me to the idea of the importance of the individual response to listening to music within therapy and how it should be chosen, if possible, by the patient. I am fascinated that you write that when you listen to music you become it with your entire being. And in *Music Therapy in Context* you write 'Music is not about the person – it is the person'. It would seem that a process of identification happens within listening too.

Mercedes: I am thinking about improvisation here, which is a bit different from listening. We usually use the word 'identification' in terms of 'identification with', don't we, which implies a separateness between the I and the identified other. So the other remains outside oneself. And I am thinking about improvi-sation in music therapy because improvisation is a bit different from listening . . . so it's almost using music as a vehicle for . . . finding various bits of myself.

MB: Yes . . . Self-therapy as it is sometimes called.

Mercedes: I think that's what happens sometimes in improvisation because one is creating and co-creating. It is a mutual process. There is feedback because when I start to play, that impacts on me in a kind of ongoing loop of authenticity with the client. It has to feel really authentic to me and also to the client.

MB: Is it a feeling of authenticity rather than a cognitive thought?

Mercedes: Yes it is a feeling. It is an ongoing process of becoming . . . of being becomed, if that's possible?

MB: Yes.

Mercedes: It is a process of being shaped, being formed. So in a sense when I hear a music therapy recording, and even now when I listen to work I've done 20 years ago, I remember with absolute clarity the music and the person. I remember the moment, the music, the person . . . I know him!

MB: You know that moment?

Mercedes: I know the moment and I also know the person and I know myself and that person.

MB: Mmn. Yes.

Mercedes: And I think that's a sensate experience. It's not just a memory of remembering.

MB: A kind of parallel is when a patient comes into the room talking about a piece of music she has heard that has associations with different important people and events in her life and these associations are tactile, the felt material of a coat or the colour of a dress.

Mercedes: The music was a vehicle for gathering an event that you worked on.

MB: Yes, that's right . . . but I don't think that this would have worked if I had been outside the music . . . I had to be in the music with her.

Mercedes: Ah . . .

MB: And know . . . know from the inside the texture of that feeling, if you like.

Mercedes: So it's about the music . . . always being in a context.

MB: Of course . . . of course. That is the title of one of your books.

Mercedes: And there is of course GIM (Guided Imagery and Music). These practitioners are very skilled at using music in particular ways.

MB: But practitioners of GIM actually choose the music, don't they, which is a bit different from what I'm talking about.

Mercedes: It is, however, an informed choice . . . but there is always a question about imposing.

MB: Yes . . . but I can understand there may be times when the client or patient is not in a place to make choices at all. You write about 'becoming the music', becoming the energy. This sounds more an experience of feeling than of distinct emotions or feelings. What is this deep flowing feeling? Can you say a bit more about it?

Mercedes: I use the word energy and I don't know if I want to give it another name . . . because energy has such multiple meanings. We were discussing the Grand National the other day and the energy of those horses, the power and the momentum, and the sort of gathering in order to leap, and the rise in tension, and the resolution as you land with a thump . . . and then you go on. That is an amazing example of momentum and waiting and intensity and phrasing.

And it is not only the movement, it is also what that sort of energy does to the air around it. It's how it is displaced . . . I was watching a video of Ellen MacArthur in that amazing boat . . . and how she worked with the energy of the sea and its power. And how this engagement displaces things around it. And when I hear music I hear pure energy . . . energy in sound . . . I don't really want to give it any other name. I've also just thought of energy in terms of how it collects people. I was in Edinburgh at a traditional folk music festival and it was a very intimate space, maybe 150 people, and a little stage. We were in the front row and three musicians were playing traditional folk music in a very intelligent way . . . very fresh . . . and it had infinite possibilities for the unexpected. I was very aware of how there were times when I started cranking up the energy of the music and people around us started tapping their toes . . . and the performers would collect this even more and then suddenly release it and then everyone would quieten down again . . . I don't think they were doing it in a manipulative way but when energy is around and allowed to permeate the group then people are gathered in it and go with it . . . contribute to it. It is highly spontaneous . . . the music is organised but there are possibilities for the unexpected.

MB: Yes, yes . . . leaving it open.

Mercedes: And afterwards there was a Swedish group, but they were almost too polished, leaving very few possibilities in terms of participation in the energy.

MB: It is interesting that you don't listen to music after your yoga class.

Mercedes: I think that's linked to the energy. I know what yoga does to *my* energy . . . because I have a lot of head energy, so I can spin in my head . . . and what yoga does is ground me . . . reconnects me to the earth and rebalances me. I know it sounds new-ageish, but I don't know how else to put it. So after the yoga, the last one, the death pose . . . I think I die every time . . . I think it is a preparation for death actually. I am very, very still . . . and I don't want to be disturbed.

MB: This is almost happening just now isn't it. I am trying to be in energetic conversation and it's almost as if you are slowing down . . . breathing quietly . . . and almost disappearing . . . which is interesting in itself . . . so there is a stillness that must be respected.

Mercedes: Yes.

MB: Until you are ready to move on again.

Mercedes: Mmn.

MB: Is there a gathering of energy afterwards?

Mercedes: Yes . . . just becoming very still . . . but then I usually get into my car and drive. So I do need to re-engage. It's not a remote stillness . . . but it's just a coming down and re-entering . . . but I definitely don't want music.

MB: You write that home is not a particularly good place for listening to music as you and your partner have very different musical tastes. This suggests that your choice of music is deeply important for you?

Mercedes talked about herself and her partner who is a musician and composes and arranges music and how she is very sensitive to what music is around. They have very different musical tastes, her partner being a brass instrumentalist, and how it is often brass music she listens to and how brass music is frequently big and full and just too much. To manage this Mercedes knows that her partner listens when she is not around, so that's fine. But music is deeply important for both of them and Simon Frith's phrase about music filling a space was mentioned. Mercedes observed that music can be invasive and how she needs to be sensitive about invading common space with *her* music. We then talked about all the music that is around us; the never-ending invasion of music from shops, cars, telephones. Mercedes recalled an underground station in Brussels and loud rock-type music coming from a public loudspeaker and also the Heathrow Express in this country with its 'busy loud descending swooping sounds'. We wondered about what that does to human ears after a long flight . . . and about the public invasion of personal space.

I then asked Mercedes about her earliest musical experiences.

Mercedes: I'm not sure that I have an earliest musical memory as such but I've been told stories about myself when I was very young so I'm not sure what's a memory or a story I have been told. But I've been told that when I was a toddler my mum noticed that when we came home from Church I'd go and sit on the rocking horse and sing whatever hymns we had sung and I used to sing very accurately and she thought Ah! . . . I think that made her realise that maybe music ought to be explored in some way. Then I recall being at a school in Italy and a wonderful piano teacher who seemed to be very fond of her because she used to give her piggy-back rides to the room on the main floor where she had her lesson. I was brought up in the French tradition and learning Sol-feg (Sol-fah) every morning after breakfast. This was along with nursery rhymes. There was also a piano teacher in her teens who was ghastly!

MB: Mmn . . . (some shared laughter). You write about Mass in St Peter's. What did it mean for you then?

Mercedes: With the Pope dying recently I've been thinking about it a lot and I'm not sure if I can separate the music from the entire spectacle . . . the entire effect. It was always such a big event . . . St Peter's is a big place especially if you're small . . . and there were always lots of people. It was something like belonging to the tribe. I had a sense of being part of the collective or something greater . . . I don't think that's what I thought at the time . . . but looking back . . . what it meant then was . . . singing. Because I sang in the choir the meaning was always couched in music and preparing music for a Mass . . . I sang in a children's choir so it was tied up with the performance . . . the rehearsals . . . the activity of singing. Of course there were the interminable services in Latin and also you fasted so you were hungry . . . yes time was slow . . . but there was also the focus of singing. That's energising in itself.

But it wasn't just attending Mass, it was being part of . . . it was also a social experience. It was also a bit competitive. I remember one service when there was a French children's choir across the aisle and I remember thinking whether their singing was better than ours or were we better than them. There was also collective passion. It was a big event when the Pope used to come. All the people clapped way over the top . . . I remember that . . . the sudden *frisson* of excitement.

I then enquired where Mercedes studied music and found that she had really studied all her life. First in Italy and then in South Africa where she studied it at university. She also studied psychology. She recalled that originally she wanted to be a performer and found music at university quite boring. It was a very repressive time in South Africa. There was apartheid and the students on her campus were very active and radical in Johannesburg. There was a heavy presence of the military and the police. She takes up her story.

Mercedes: I kept thinking what am I doing studying music in the middle of what's going on in this country? In my fourth year I went walking in the mountains with some student friends from Cape Town. One was a medic doing an internship and she talked of there being all these therapies in the hospital. I asked if they had music and she replied 'Oh yes . . . music therapy'. And as she said those words the penny dropped. Her words really spoke to me.

MB: So just a chance meeting.

Mercedes: But nothing is ever by chance . . . but yes, a chance meeting.

MB: Mmn . . . so there is no family music?

Mercedes: Oh no! Not at all.

MB: So that is how you chose music therapy as a career?

Mercedes: I went to South America as a student observer to the World Congress of Music Therapy in Buenos Aires and I listened to all these music therapists and I thought this was a load of rubbish. I knew nothing about it but I thought this is *not* what I want to do. They are mad. I was 20 and had a very negative response. So I said to myself 'forget it'. So I came back and did a bit of teaching. But a friend of mine gave me a pamphlet and said I should go to this talk by another music therapist, Julienne Cartwright. And when I heard this woman I said, 'This is what I want to do. This is what I've been waiting for'. This was it.

MB: But how was this experience different from what you heard at the World Congress?

Mercedes: It felt utterly genuine and authentic, not put on, not a performance. When I was at the Congress in South America there seemed to be a hysteria about 'Oh those poor children – and what can we do for them'. So after I listened to Julienne, I introduced myself to her and she became my mentor in fact.

We moved on to talk about improvisational music therapy and how it is about active improvisation between client and therapist and how the technique resonates with early infant/mother engagement where mother responds atten-tively to the sounds and gestures of the baby. I then wondered if Mercedes held the view that through this process the therapist attunes to the client and draws him or her further into a dynamic feeling relationship.

Mercedes: To begin to answer this . . . it is definitely the music *between* the therapist and the client that is the technique resonating with the early infant/ mother relationship. It is like the mother/baby relationship but it is also different. In the early infant/mother relationship the baby doesn't really have a choice about how to engage – because the baby doesn't yet have language. So the mother adapts to motherese [coo-ing and babbling *MB*]. In order to engage she exaggerates the prosody of her encounter but extends it. And there is also this business of mismatching at times, and sometimes the therapist has to draw away. It is not just a dynamic feeling relationship, it is a dynamic feeling relationship and a musical relationship. I don't know that you can separate the two; they are the same. Also in music therapy we come with our own social world and different musicking languages if you like and there is this delicate balance between the genres almost overriding the communication. What I mean is that in the improvisation I might get a musical idea and often it is not an interpersonal musical idea. I might start improvising an Irish jig and you have to be careful because there are times when you might suddenly lose the client. In other words you might begin playing music instead of co-creating with the client.

MB: Yes, the empathy suffers here . . . would you say there is a difference between therapists who use words and music and the therapist who works solely in music?

Mercedes: My take on this is that the whole debate is that words and music or music alone is sort of either/or thinking and that the debate has really moved on. This is not talked about now. The problem of whether one used words or not was confused with whether one was working psychodynamically or not. The debate then became polarised into whether one was using a music-centred approach that was caricatured as working only in music or the psychodynamic approach that said that working in music was not enough, you had to have words to bring insight. You can work psychodynamically in words or you cannot work psychodynamically in either . . . it is not linked to the medium. It is linked to how you want to work. I think it has all ground to a halt now and we've moved on. For myself I tend to think neurologically now, really activating the body, the being, the mind, . . . activating the person. If you are going to use Winnicott or Trevarthen it's going to be about what frame of knowledge helps to make sense of the work.

MB: So who are the neurological thinkers who underpin your work?

Mercedes: Oh Trevarthen, Malloch and communicative musicality because this is really at the heart of my understanding of what we do and how we do it. So improvisation activates my communicative musicality as well as the client's. It's activated through conversation, and it's activated through musicking. But musicking uses genres and idioms, different cultural modes of being-in-relationship and these all spark each other off. I found Winnicott's views useful earlier in my work but I don't find them very useful at the moment. What I do find useful is communicative musicality . . . of moving in sympathy with the client, of sharing mind states, sharing the experience of time and co-creating a time experience. I think that any experience has a particular quality or hue surrounding it that remains with us and we kind of live it. I find this when listening to opera. If we start talking about it immediately afterwards we can close it before the experience is finished. When we start talking, language and discourse starts reframing the experience.

MB: Has the experience of music changed for you over the years?

Mercedes: Oh the experience of music changes all the time for me. I do less clinical work now. I'm running a training programme so I'm doing much more listening now than when I was practising and that's a different experience. I tend not to go to live concerts because I live in South Africa where there aren't that many. Because my listening is often linked to my work I would say that for the last ten years I listen to world music rather than classical music, which I rarely listen to now. I will go to live concerts of classical music when they come up but other than that I rarely listen to it. Partly because it's too big . . . I listen when I'm driving and that's not conducive to big works.

MB: So tell me about world music.

Mercedes: I listen to Latin American, traditional music, folk music from other countries. I've got CDs of gypsy music for instance . . . and I am also on the lookout for other genres for the students to alert them to different ways of playing. When I was in Brittany I went straight to the CD shop because I wanted to know about the local music and what people played in Brittany. It's all to do with being *in situ* . . . being there. What music does this place have? What do the people play? What are its musical roots? Living in South Africa I listen to a radio programme on a Saturday called *The African Connection* and it plays musical genres from all over the Continent . . . a fantastic programme.

MB: May I ask more personally where you are now with music? If it was taken away from you what would that mean for you?

Mercedes: Oh I'd be dead . . . no question. It's part of being alive. I'd never be without music . . . no question.

MB: You can't even imagine . . .?

Mercedes: No. It's not a possibility . . . not imaginable.

MB: What is the most important piece of music for you and what does it mean for you?

Mercedes: I can't answer that question. It's completely dependent on the mood I'm in at the moment . . . what I'm doing. There's no piece of music I would say is the most important . . . no.

MB: So you're really a world musician now?

Mercedes: Oh I don't know if that means I'm a world musician . . . I can't answer that question . . . it's the wrong question.

MB: It's the wrong question?

Mercedes: For me.

MB: What is the right question for you?

Mercedes: I think . . . What would I like to listen to right now and why? That would be it. But I think about a recent event and remember what I thought then. I remember the death of Pope John Paul II and I remember thinking about the Brahms' *Requiem* . . . it works for me like that . . . I wouldn't choose that piece today.

MB: What would you say today?

Mercedes: I think I'm feeling a bit speedy . . . a bit upbeat, a bit panicky because I've got a lot to do. I think I would listen to something quite fast and upbeat . . . and panicky really (some shared laughter). I might listen to some music from a fantastic Chilean group called Inti-Illimani. So you see how I can't answer your previous question. One day it's the Brahms' *Requiem* and on another it's Inti-Illimani. It depends on the situation.

MB: Thank you very much Mercedes.

Mercedes: You're very welcome.

CHAPTER 2

Conversation with Katie Melua

Katie Melua is a contemporary singer and this interview was different from the others. It was not face-to-face as it was not possible to meet up with Katie due to her heavy commitments, so Katie very kindly offered to have a telephone conversation with me on what music means for her.

MB: Hello Katie, so nice of you to ring. I'll go over a little bit of your history but you can tell me more about yourself as we talk.

Katie: OK.

MB: You were born in Georgia in 1984 and then you moved to Moscow.

Katie: Well, we lived in Moscow for a year or so when I was very, very young but we lived in Georgia until I was about eight.

MB: But I read some somewhere that there was some memory when you were in Moscow about pancakes. Is that right?

Katie: Oh yeah . . . well, it's just a funny little thing that I remembered about Moscow. It was that there were pancakes everywhere. I was only about three at the time.

MB: But you went back to Georgia to the seaside town of Batcheme?

Katie: Yeah, yeah.

MB: And then you came to Ireland when you were about eight or nine . . . because your father took up a post there as a heart surgeon.

Katie: Yes, that's right. Then after living in Belfast for five years his contract came to an end and we moved to south London where he took up a post and the whole family moved as well.

MB: Do you have any musical memories of your time in Russia . . . does anything special come to mind?

Katie: When you say Russia I think you're including Georgia as well. Georgia was part of the USSR but it became independent in 1991 and I do have lots of memories about Georgia. That's when I really started singing. Georgia is a very artistic cultural place and nearly everyone sings there or plays the piano. I remember that the electricity used to go off in the winter time and by way of entertainment my mum would play the piano and we would put on little concerts at home. Yes I have a lot of memories. That was when I first began singing lessons at seven or eight and she was a really brilliant teacher. When I go back to Georgia I still see her and try to have some singing lessons from her. Her name is Mzia.

MB: Do you remember songs from then?

Katie: Oh yes, a lot of Georgian popular songs . . . and I used to sing duets which was great.

MB: You moved to Ireland when you were nine. What music were you aware of at that time?

Katie: Well, I had heard Madonna and Michael Jackson in Georgia, but coming to Belfast it was like coming into a different world. I think Boy Bands had just started . . . I had Georgian popular music behind me, and also Georgian folk music. I can also remember hearing Georgian male voice choir singing and they had 8-part harmony!

MB: So you brought all that experience of listening with you to Ireland?

Katie: No not really . . . this is the music I left behind, if you like. Because I was so young I hadn't really gotten into the folk music of Georgia but every time I went back, there was that experience of re-discovery. But in Belfast the music suddenly switched to the pop charts and I was also introduced to Irish folk music at the Catholic school I went to.

MB: Your brother went to a Protestant school and you went to a Catholic one, which was quite a deliberate choice by your parents?

Katie: Yeah, yeah.

MB: What did you want to be when you were about thirteen or fourteen?

Katie: Music was really like a nice hobby for me at that time. I really enjoyed school, especially history lessons, and at the time I really didn't think about becoming a singer. I hadn't really made up my mind.

MB: But by the time you were thirteen or fourteen you must have been singing quite a lot because you won a TV talent competition?

Katie: Well . . . I was singing quite a bit . . . if you remember I had had singing lessons in Georgia but it was still a hobby and when I went in for that talent competition . . . I don't know if you ever heard of it . . . it was a children's competition called 'Stars up their Nose'. It wasn't quite 'Stars in their Eyes', not anything really that serious.

MB: Anyway, you won it!

Katie: Yeah, for a fourteen-year-old it was great and I got a makeover worth £250.

MB: And were you nervous when you sang?

Katie: Yeah of course . . . but, as I said before, even at that stage I really hadn't decided what I wanted to do.

MB: You went on to the Brit School of Performing Arts where you did A-level music. When did you start writing songs Katie?

Katie: It started about the year before I went to the Brit School, when I was about fifteen or sixteen. That was suddenly when music became something I definitely wanted to do as a career.

MB: So it's when you started writing you began to think of music as a career?

Katie: I started writing but I also got a computer with music recording software and it was really nice for home video. I had a keyboard which I had had for many years and I bought a mike and stuff and so I not only started writing at that age, I started recording my own stuff . . . and I was quite impressed with it. So every waking hour I had was in my room writing and making recordings. That was when the sort of hobby became something I definitely wanted to do as a career. I didn't know at that point whether I wanted to be a singer or not. But I knew I definitely wanted to be involved with music and it didn't really matter what. And then I went to Brit School and did the music A-level.

   It was really a good course because not only did it deal with everything about music, listening, theory, etc., but you had to perform every month. But what was really interesting for me on this course was that it covered music technology and I wanted to learn a bit about that.

MB: Now you say that originality is important for you in music. Could you say a bit more about that?

Katie: When I say originality is the most important thing, I remember at the Brit course I really enjoyed the first year and the musical genres of R&B (rhythm and blues) and hip hop and that was fine at the time, but as I began to know other musicians and discover what they did and have teachers who were very passionate about music and discovering artists like the Beatles, Led Zeppelin, Ella Fitzgerald . . . discovering a real cross-section of artists, I began to feel that the music in the pop charts wasn't really of the same standard. It wasn't the same standard that it had been 30 years before.

MB: That's interesting.

Katie: I was quite sad about it . . . and then I came across Eva Cassidy.

MB: Now tell me what was great about this.

Katie: I didn't know anything about her and I just heard this voice and I remember exactly where I was. I was in a car coming back to Brighton from London. My mum was driving and she had made a 'Now' compilation of songs on a tape. She had recorded pretty much all of the sad CDs and suddenly Eva's voice came on. The tape ran out half way through *Over the Rainbow*, but there was just something about the voice . . . a cry of emotion . . . and her voice was crystal clear . . . almost angelic. It was what she was doing with her voice that was so original and how she reached me as a listener at an emotional level. I then tried to analyse how she made small changes in the song to bring about this effect. For instance, in the original classic song there is a leap between the tones on the word 'Somewhere' (over the rainbow) and she changed this so that 'Somewhere' was on the same note. This tiny change seemed to make the song completely her own. That's a really original touch. She just had a way of singing songs as if she had written them herself.

MB: Very personal to her.

Katie: Yes . . . we'd all heard them before but not sung like that. It was as if she'd shone a different light on them.

MB: Yes that's very interesting . . . and perhaps you feel that you would like to be that kind of artist?

Katie: Well I don't think that anyone could replace Eva or try to imitate what she did. I think she was completely her own self. But it's more about the effect on me when I listen to Eva. It's that kind of experience in the listener that I think I strive for, that ability to reach someone so powerfully. That's what makes a great artist for me.

MB: Can you give us an example of how Eva Cassidy affected your work?

Katie: After I heard Eva Cassidy a whole kind of thing happened for me in my songwriting. I picked up the guitar, and this is only about three or four years ago, and this song came out and I started writing from *playing* the guitar. I usually wrote on the computer and I found that the songs I was writing from playing the guitar were different. Because I only had the guitar and my voice, *that* was what I could work on.

MB: There was no machine between.

Katie: There was no machine, no computer with the plethora of effects available. When I wrote at the computer I would want to try out the drum track slowly, for example, so that would distract me. So instead of finishing the melody, the lyrics and the chord structures, which I think now is an essential to a good song, I was excited and distracted by all these effects. But when I was writing from the guitar I had got down to the essentials . . . the lyrics, the harmony and the melody. A lot of music is all about rhythm from a computer and only about rhythm. When you listen to R&B music it's all about rhythm, it's about making the body move. This is not a bad thing at all . . . but what I was discovering was a different focal point.

MB: That's right.

Katie: So . . . although this is a matter of taste, what makes a good song for me is all three, the melody, the harmony and the lyrics. They have to be amazing, because they are the stem of the song. That's what will survive in 100 years.

MB: Yes, . . . you write that you are influenced by Irish folk song and Indian music. What is your favourite Irish folk song?

Katie: Oh I think *Danny Boy*. It has the bending of the note, which I love in Irish folk song. Enya, who is a very contemporary artist . . . I think that a lot of her appeal is rooted in Irish folk song. Her music has a very celtic flavour, a pure sound . . . it's very difficult to describe. Talking about music here is like trying to taste a recipe from a cook book.

MB: Yes, that's right. But can you tell me what it is about *Danny Boy* that you particularly like?

Katie: It's the nostalgia of it. I love Belfast, so music reminds me of my time in Ireland and I love going back there. The people are so warm and kind and there is a really nice spirit. I think this song for some reason seems to capture that.

MB: Yes indeed, it's a lovely melody. Can I turn to Indian music for a moment? Can you say what appeals to you most about this?

Katie: I guess what appeals to me most is the rhythm. Indian music has this body rhythm. I think it's quite close to Georgian music in this sense. The Georgian drums are quite similar to those in Indian music and the rhythms are not straight 4/4 for instance.

MB: It really moves.

Katie: It really moves and changes all the time in the dancing. For example, the men dance with knives and it's very exciting. The rhythms are very exciting as there are a lot of off-beats and cross rhythms. I think that's the connection with Indian music.

MB: Yes that's quite fascinating . . . I would like to talk about some songs now that you have recorded Katie and in particular *Far Away Voice* which is dedicated to Eva Cassidy. Can you tell us a bit more about this song?

Katie: Well it's quite strange you ask about this song because it's the song I wrote when I first composed with the guitar instead of the computer. As I said earlier, if you look at the guitar part it's incredibly simple, and maybe that's because it was the first song I composed like that. But I first heard her voice on that car journey from Brighton to London and other than that I knew nothing about her . . . I just heard this voice and I was captivated. I didn't even bother to read the record sleeve. I said to my boyfriend that we must go and hear this girl live because she's absolutely amazing. I knew she was a new artist because I had never heard anyone like her before. She sounded very young as well . . . so there was no reason for me to presume she was no longer alive. But he then said that she had died a few years ago and that was hard for me to take in. Here was this singer that I could really admire and she was not alive anymore. So all these emotions really inspired this song. It came out very quickly. There are songs that you write on a quick impulse to an emotional feeling . . . you almost don't have to think about it and that was how this song was.

There are other songs that I do think about quite carefully . . . when I want to tell a story. But when I began to think of Eva . . . Mmn . . . yes, . . . I was quite shocked when I began to read more about her. She had never really been famous when she was alive. She used to play all the time around her local bars and people enjoyed her singing a lot but she never really ended up getting signed up to a record company.

But this song *Far Away Voice* isn't only about her specifically – it's also about my generation. And it's almost being born at a time when I don't feel it was the best from a listening point of view. I so wish for instance that I had been at the first Beatles concerts or I wish that I had seen Joni Mitchell when she started or Jimi Hendrix. So this song is really about the sadness of not having heard these people and a sadness for my generation. I felt quite angry at times but as I've developed in my career I've discovered that there are amazing artists today but they're not mainstream. You've just got to find them.

MB: Now in this song *Far Away Voice* it's as if someone is calling beyond the grave and you sort of join in with them in a kind of 'whoo' sound?

Katie: Yes, in the song is a crying out and it's different for every listener. For me I think it's about wanting her to be alive.

MB: Yes, it's very moving and evocative, 'Are you over the hill?' and 'Do you think people listen?'

Katie: I mean I really wonder if somewhere she realises that so much of her is left behind and treasured by so many people . . . as any artist will tell you, the greatest ambition for any true artist is to have their music live on beyond their death.

MB: That way you have a sort of immortality.

Katie: Yes, you are immortal in a sense and, yes, the song incorporates that as well.

MB: We were talking about Irish songs earlier and I wonder if there is an Irish influence in this song?

Katie: No I don't think so on a conscious level but I spent quite a lot of my life there and it's completely possible that an Irish sound surfaced in this song, but it was not really something that was going on in my conscious mind when I was writing it.

MB: Another great song that you sing is of course *The Closest Thing to Crazy* and I feel that its huge appeal has something to do with the fact that most people have felt those kinds of feelings about someone at some time in their lives.

Katie: Absolutely . . . I mean most of the great songs have captured a powerful feeling that is general and has been experienced by most people.

I felt really happy when I discovered this song because Mike Batt had written it many years before. Mike had recorded it himself as a solo artist and basically he had put it on an album of his and it had never got released, for political reasons . . . whatever. We had experimental sessions listening to songs that I had written and songs that he had written. On one particular session he was playing something from this album and I didn't think it was quite right for what we were doing. I had the sleeve notes of the album in my hand and I read *The Closest Thing to Crazy* . I asked what this one was and he said 'Oh that's an old song, I don't think that'll be right for you'. But I played it and I said 'Come on Mike, we've got to record it, it's such a brilliant song.' I felt it was a classic straight away and that I had heard it many times before, even though I hadn't . . . you know what I mean?

MB: Yes, it had a shape and a feel about it you knew from somewhere.

Katie: Yes, there was something very familiar about it. I asked him to record it and he said 'OK then!' It was really funny and we laugh about it now but right up until the last moment he was unsure of it. It was my Dad who said 'This is such a great song you should certainly keep it'. It was the radio then that picked it as a single and then the public.

MB: It's really about giving your heart to someone completely who then breaks it . . . isn't it?

Katie: Yes, I certainly view that song like that. But again it's a song that never really satisfies the particular situation. It's really about being on the edge in a relationship, when you're not really able to be yourself with the person you're with. Something's not quite right. It could be a happy relationship but you're so happy you alienate everyone else around you . . . that sometimes happens.

MB: Yes – it could be all of those things.

Katie: Yes, exactly.

MB: Now, how does this song really work musically do you think? There are, for instance, two verses of questions, and then there is the rise and fall of each line. Then there is the awful realisation that you are losing your mind to this person. There is then a build-up of tension followed by the violins coming in with a lovely counterpoint and the feeling of warmth with the whole orchestra and then it is repeated.

Katie: Yes that's true and for me there are the 3/4 and 4/4 passages which kind of clash . . . but it works.

MB: Turning to another song that you yourself have written called *Belfast*. Can you tell us something about that?

Katie: This song is really about this great city and I suppose it is like a lot of places where there is political instability. People who have never been there think of it as dangerous and they would never go there. But taking this view, you don't really think of the human families there who try to get on with their everyday lives and struggle through . . . trying to live normal lives and be happy on a certain level.

This is quite an expressive song and I guess I try to talk about the daily life I saw. It was like I saw the *shadow* of the 'troubles' because I never spoke to anyone directly about them. For instance you would see something painted on the walls in Irish and you would think you were looking at a cartoon, but it was a man holding a gun. You would have to put this image alongside me as an eight- or nine-year-old going to school and having a really great time everyday . . . but experiencing all this atmosphere and remembering it.

MB: These were very unusual circumstances for you and when you write about the 'limited freedom to fly' . . ., these would be the penguins or people who could not easily remove themselves from the situation.

Katie: Yes exactly . . . and the cats obviously . . .

MB: The dying that went on . . .

Katie: And not analysing it too much – they say cats have nine lives, but they don't really . . . . This song was also about my understanding of the 'troubles' and how the conflict wasn't really about religion. One of the main differences between the Catholics and Protestants, as I saw it, was not that they attached more importance to the Virgin Mary, it was about whether Northern Ireland remained part of the United Kingdom or not. It was really about who rules Northern Ireland.

MB: And you write about the paintings on the walls being 'no motif'. But they were meaningful?

Katie: Yes absolutely . . . it's another form of art. It's someone expressing himself in a political context.

MB: Yes, that's right . . . going back for a moment to the cats dying nine times. There's a very circular locked-in feeling when the music accompanies these words. I'm wondering if you remember such feelings when you were writing it. It's just going on and on . . . and it's happening over and over.

Katie: Yes, I would say that's not something I was completely aware of. It was more a play on words as I remember it and people do have only nine lives here. It's dark what happened . . . it's about death.

MB: Have you got some new songs ready to be brought out, Katie?

Katie: Yes, there are some new ones and we will just have to see if people like them. We'll see, we'll see.

MB: This is a rather hard question now Katie . . . what if music was to be taken away from you . . .what would you imagine that would be like?

Katie: Oh . . . I think that feels impossible for me. The only way I could put myself in that place is if suddenly I lost my hearing and my voice. But it's not such an important part of my life that I would lose a sense of existence as well. I sometimes think of life as a movie and music as the sound track if you like.

MB: So the sound track is perhaps the sound track to who you are?

Katie: Yes, absolutely . . . but I *really* can't imagine myself in that situation at all. Having no music is something I can't really imagine.

MB: So you really identify with music?

Katie: Yes . . . I love the crazy process. There's nothing like having written a song. It's just the most amazing thing in the world.

MB: Katie, I really want to thank you very much for making time to have this conversation. At the moment you are dashing to another engagement by car and we are having this conversation on the telephone.

Katie: It's been really great talking to you.

MB: Thanks again Katie, and good luck with your new album.

CHAPTER 3

Conversation with Baroness Julia Neuberger

Baroness Neuberger is a Rabbi and writer on public issues.

MB: How do you experience music, Julia? Do you go with the flow or do you listen to particular music?

Baroness Neuberger: It depends what the music is. I almost always listen to classical music . . . occasionally jazz. And I suppose what I would have to say is it depends on how well I know the piece . . . it depends on why I'm playing music. I listen to music a great deal and I do the thing that everybody tells you you shouldn't do . . . I listen to music when I work.

  If I'm writing something I listen to music . . . and there I am aware that I use it almost as a distraction. So there's one thing going on outside that blocks out other distractions.

MB: So it gathers your concentration?

Baroness Neuberger: It gathers my concentration. If I'm writing something of any length, particularly if I'm writing part of a book I will *always* have music going on. What's really awful and all musicologists will hate me for saying this . . . I quite often play the same thing again and again and again. It almost doesn't matter much what it is, provided it's familiar.

MB: So what would it be?

Baroness Neuberger: Well I mean . . . at various points it would be the Brahms *Requiem* again and again . . . it has been *Tosca* or it has been *Turandot* or it has been *Rigoletto* . . . it's got to be familiar. It's got to be music I really love so that I don't have to keep disentangling it. I suppose I'm reasonably musical, so what I would do if I'm listening to something new would be that I'd spend quite a lot of time disentangling it in my head so that it's become familiar, and when it's familiar then I will use it . . . as an exclusion of all other distractions I suppose. It will have become something I know well so it's echoing in my head and it concentrates my thoughts.

MB: And you can relax into it?

Baroness Neuberger: I relax into it.

MB: Now would you say that you are captured by the emotional plot?

Baroness Neuberger: Can I say something a bit different here? When I'm listening to something relatively new or something I know less well then first of all I'm absolutely captured by the emotion. If it's opera . . . then obviously . . . but if it's a symphony, I'm quite interested in the plot of the music . . . it tells a story. It's both an intellectual story and an emotional story. That's why music is so powerful.

If you take something like the Bach *Brandenburg Concertos*, which I listen to quite a lot . . . I can't listen to them as a distraction because I always spend my time disentangling the various parts in my head – so that's intellectually and emotionally uplifting.

MB: They almost compel attention?

Baroness Neuberger: So they compel attention . . . so I can't use them for background music. I can use other equally great works but they are different . . . like the Brahms *Requiem* . . . like the great Italian operas. I know them very well and I know the stories so they don't require me to disentangle them in the same way. They don't play to the intellect in quite the same way as Bach does.

MB: Yes, I was thinking that because you mention what we call romantic music.

Baroness Neuberger: Yes . . . I tend to listen to the romantics for distraction as well as loving them and listening to them for pleasure anyway. And if I listen to intellectual music it tends to be, for me on the whole, earlier music . . . not all, but a lot of earlier music. It would certainly be Bach . . . some Handel . . . it might be Purcell. I find that grips the intellect and I find it quite hard to relax into. There's no sweep . . . no sweep of movement that just carries me away.

MB: You've got to attend.

Baroness Neuberger: I've got to listen.

MB: Where were you born, Julia, and where did you live as a small child?

Baroness Neuberger: I was born in London and lived in London. I played a musical instrument, the violin, although my parents didn't want me to. If you look over there, there is a violin. My husband bought me a new violin for my 50th birthday. I haven't played it much and I don't play very well. I'm really at the level I was when I started when I was 8.

MB: You have to really practise the violin.

Baroness Neuberger: Well you have to practise and you have to have lessons so I've got to get my act together . . . but I did play . . . I played in the school orchestra. I played occasionally for an opera. I'd really love to play and I'm really bad! (shared laughter).

MB: Are there any memories of music associated with your early years?

Baroness Neuberger: Well I suppose a lot of the music from my early years would have been at the Synagogue as a child. So a lot of it would have been liturgical music of a particular Jewish variety. So it would have been very good organ music, which is not typical of some Jewish music. It would have been singing very traditional songs at the end of the service, it would have been a very fine choir, the West London Synagogue Choir . . . so that would have been part of my experience. But when I got older although quite little still, I was very musical as a child, and my mother was not. My father was musical but sort of blanked it out and they didn't listen to music really . . . so I was beating them up to let me go to the Robert Mayer concerts. But these concerts were on Saturday mornings when we went to the Synagogue so I had to do a deal with my father so that I could go to these concerts provided I went to the Synagogue every other Saturday.

MB: Can you tell me a little about the Robert Mayer concerts?

Baroness Neuberger: Well the Robert Mayer concerts were completely inspirational. I absolutely adored them. He was an extraordinary man. I went with a school group and I just remember these concerts introduced me to the intellectual part of music because what I learned was how to disentangle . . . .

MB: You've used that word in connection with music before.

Baroness Neuberger: Yes, if you grew up in a house where old 78s were played and nobody told you how a symphony works, how the orchestra works, everything was a bit of a tangle . . . but all became clearer when music like the *Young Person's Guide to the Orchestra* (Benjamin Britten) was explained . . . or listening to one movement of a symphony and somebody taking the trouble to tell you what's going on was great. Occasionally there would be chamber music and you would hear the different parts separately and then you would hear them played together . . . that was the thing that tipped me over into getting hooked.

MB: What about music at school?

Baroness Neuberger: Yes . . . I played at school and I listened quite a lot at school but that was quite different somehow. It was more relaxed at the Robert Mayer concerts and they were certainly longer. They were about an hour and a bit I suppose, so you had long enough to really soak it up. They had very good programmes and they taught you about crescendos, for example, and they told you a lot in a way that programme notes don't. They really got you to think about different aspects of music such as the composer's life. I used to read these *Lives of the Great Composers* all the time when I was a kid.

MB: Was it the person of Mayer who really brought this about?

Baroness Neuberger: No, in a sense he left them to get on with it . . . to produce the concerts . . . he said what he wanted. But they knew the children needed a knowledge base. Then there was the playing to the emotions and the intellect as you learnt about the story. You learnt about romantic music . . . you learnt about the passionate in music but you also learnt about the intellectual rigour in putting it together. I think *that* was very clever. I think it was quite an intellectual approach to people who were very young. I think I was 8 or 9 when I first went . . . quite little.

MB: Are there any persons in your family you particularly associate with music?

Baroness Neuberger: Well . . . my father more than my mother. My father bought my mother a wonderful 'music centre', you would call it, when she was 75 or so in 1990. But in spite of the fact that she said she wanted to listen to music, she did so fairly rarely and she always answered the phone in the room where the music was playing, so it was constantly interrupted. My father occasionally listened . . . he was much more musical. We took him to the opera sometimes. I think he really didn't explore his own musical interest and when he was in hospital a lot towards the end of his life, we got him a 'Walkman' and lots of tapes and he listened then . . . particularly to Brahms.

MB: I would like to talk about music and hospitals a bit more but going back to school for a moment . . . are there musical memories from there?

Baroness Neuberger: Yes . . . a most wonderful music teacher who is still alive, a Miss Jean Middlemiss. If it hadn't been for her I don't think I would have got in to music at all and I am eternally grateful. I think she recognised that I was more interested than most. I did music theory to grade 5 just because I wanted to know how it worked . . . music more so than scientific things . . . I was never very interested in those!

MB: What did you listen to as a teenager?

Baroness Neuberger: I listened to the Beatles and I listened to the 'Singing Nun' Dominique and the first sort of 'pop' record I had was *Summer Holiday* by Cliff Richard. Other than that I listened to classical music and I always have ever since . . . mainly opera. Anything that isn't classical music seems to be on the edge for me. And because of Robert Mayer and youth and music I went to masses of opera . . . I went to Covent Garden in the cheap seats for years.

MB: What particular piece of music were you drawn to as a young adult?

Baroness Neuberger: Well, we did Monteverdi's *Orfeo* at school and I was very drawn to that and got to know it very well. But then Bach's Brandenburg concertos were all through my teenage years as were Bach's unaccompanied 'cello suites and opera, Mozart or Italian 19th century operas. I've never liked Wagner . . . I still don't. I find some of his music compelling but I so dislike the plots, so it was mainly Italian 19th century opera.

MB: What about modern opera?

Baroness Neuberger: I don't listen to recordings . . . I go to it. For instance we're going to *1984* in a couple of weeks and we went to Tippett's *The Knot Garden* and *A Midsummer Marriage*. With modern operas you just can't listen, so I don't have recordings. What you need is the visual. One of my favourite operas is Britten's *The Turn of the Screw* . . . compelling! But you listen to it on a recording and it just doesn't do it for you.

MB: It's got to be the whole thing.

Baroness Neuberger: Yes, you've got to see the whole thing.

MB: It's almost Wagnerian in the sense that the costumes, the scenery, the music, the acting, the words, etc. have all to be experienced as a music drama.

Baroness Neuberger: Yes, in that sense. In the last production of *The Turn of the Screw* at Covent Garden everyone was on the edge of their seats. You can't do this with a recording. It's not lyrical like 19th century music.

MB: Was there a particular event in your life when music was especially important?

Baroness Neuberger: When my father was dying . . . I listened to *Dido and Aeneas* endlessly . . . endlessly. I played it when I was driving across London going from South London to the Royal Free Hospital and it still has that memory for me.

MB: That association.

Baroness Neuberger: And it was really funny because I had given him a tape of it as well, so he was listening to it and I was listening to it.

MB: That's very interesting. Something happens when two people choose to listen to music together.

Baroness Neuberger: Yes . . . but I gave it to him because it was something which was very much mine. But he listened to a lot of Mozart . . . his absolute favourite was Mozart. He listened to the symphonies, the clarinet quintet . . . partly because I gave him the tapes I knew he liked. He didn't want opera . . . he wasn't as fond of 19th century Italian as me. His father had been a Wagnerian . . . .

MB: Right . . . .

Baroness Neuberger: For many Jews, post-holocaust, Wagner has been much more difficult . . . whereas my grandfather was a German Jew who had come to England in 1906 and they were very keen Wagnerians . . . good Germans who were keen Wagnerians.

MB: How interesting.

Baroness Neuberger: They were German in a sense, not my grandfather in particular, but many of them were German Nationalists. Members of my family fought on the German side in the First World War. My father grew up being taken to a lot of Wagner but he never liked it . . . he loved Mozart. My grandfather was very musical but I didn't know him . . . he died before I was born.

MB: I note the phrase you used at the beginning about 'music and disentangling things' and this story you're telling me now almost needs to be disentangled in a way doesn't it?

Baroness Neuberger: The story about who listened to what?

MB: Yes.

Baroness Neuberger: Well, I think there is a Jewish story here. My grandparents and their families were German Jews and relatively well off, living in Frankfurt in South Germany. They were Orthodox Jews. You were an Orthodox Jew but you were also a German. Wagner expressed being German and German Nationalism from the 1870s and that was incredibly important. Anyone of their generation would have listened to quite a lot of Wagner, if they listened to music at all, and they tended to be quite cultured.

My grandfather was clearly quite musical and they did listen to music at home. Certainly my father remembered listening to Wagner as a child and he also listened to a lot of Mozart. My father played the violin in the London Conservatoire, I think that was its name, and he and his brother Harry, who was a 'cellist, used to go and play on a Sunday. They were really quite musical kids.

MB: Yes.

Baroness Neuberger: But the Wagner thing . . . I think he didn't like it because he was too young. But post-holocaust when so many of the family had died and both my grandparents were deeply involved with getting Jews out of Germany, Wagner became unappealing . . . and even Mahler, I don't terribly like. I think it's something about that period of music that is problematic and doesn't do it for me. But I think that when I found that Mime and Alberich had been deliberately turned into Jews in *Der Ring des Nibelungen* I found that pretty hard to take, and it doesn't do it for me. I don't think my father reacted as strongly as I did but he still didn't like it . . . .

MB: Returning to your writing for a moment, in your book *The Moral State We're In*, you write with real concern about the condition of some psychiatric hospitals and units and describe the work of an enlightened senior nurse in Lynfield Mount Hospital in Bradford and how he brought about real changes, one of which was banning loud music. Have you got any further thoughts about music in psychiatric hospitals?

Baroness Neuberger: Well, so many many of those old big wards, some of which still exist, you just had Radio 2, or Radio 1, or rap or whatever blasting out. If you wanted a peaceful place to get better that's absolutely hopeless. I love the idea that if people want to listen to music they've got to listen to it on headphones. And especially, if you want to have music as therapy then use it as *therapy* and be clear what you are trying to do. But just to play any old music is outrageous I think. The worst offenders are the old nursing homes and the psychogeriatric wards where they have music playing all the time, and you have people looking zomboid.

You can use music in properly thought out reminiscence therapy with older people. For example, hymns can be very effective, but often what is actually played is what the nurses want to hear . . . what's that about a therapeutic environment?! It's just as important as the visual environment. We did a lot of work on the visual environment when I was at the King's Fund but the audio is just as important. If you go round the nursing homes at the moment you see people grouped around a television set programmed to something they don't want to see.

MB: What about music in more general hospitals?

Baroness Neuberger: It's exactly the same there but one of the things that's now great, and part of the whole movement of *Arts in Health*, is live performance coming on to the ward. But opera performances and chamber music are only in the big teaching hospitals and not in the psychiatric hospitals where people are likely to be there for much longer and I think that's a real shame. But psychiatric hospitals don't have much spare cash, it's not that high up on their agenda. But clearly music is enormously valuable to many of these people. But some people need to have sound all the time. Look at supermarkets. There's always music.

MB: But doctor's surgeries are another venue with constant sound, which some people don't want.

Baroness Neuberger: It varies. Some have music and they say it keeps the patients calmer.

MB: But it depends what they play! I see difficulties about who chooses the music in the doctor's surgery or the hospital. Do you have any thoughts on this?

Baroness Neuberger: First of all people should be encouraged to put suggestions into a box. In waiting areas in Casualty this might be quite helpful, but let's have some decisions about what it is going to be. And who is going to make the decision? Not always the staff! So some positive research should be carried out. And I think that sometimes you do want silence . . . not constant music.

MB: Perhaps intense music should be avoided, pop or classical . . . and music with a strong rhythmic beat should perhaps be left out.

Baroness Neuberger: Yes, absolutely . . . it's got to be what you would have as background music.

MB: What is background music?

Baroness Neuberger: Well . . . here is a difficulty. It's got to be second rate don't you think? It's about asking people what they want and working round it. But whatever it is you don't play it so loud. Actually it should be such that you have to make an effort to hear it . . . so if you don't want to listen to it you blank it out.

MB: Returning to your own musical listening . . . do you think this has changed over the years and if so what do you retain from your earlier experience?

Baroness Neuberger: I think it's just a life-long thing. I don't know that it has changed much . . . maybe deepened. My taste has changed of course. I go to something musical a couple of times a week. We're going to the opera five times in the space of five weeks, which is a bit unusual for us . . . we don't usually manage that.

MB: What are you going to hear?

Baroness Neuberger: We went to *Un Ballo in Maschera* last week and we're going to *Madame Butterfly* and *1984* . . . I can't remember the rest. So there are lots of treats in store.

MB: Is there any one particular opera you listen to over the others?

Baroness Neuberger: Probably not. It would be mainly Verdi or Puccini . . . probably Verdi, *La Traviata* or *Rigoletto*.

MB: Can you identify what it is about *Rigoletto* that is really important for you?

Baroness Neuberger: Although it's desperately sad . . . it's got very memorable tunes. In that sense it's easy listening. It's really dramatic but if you're not really listening you might miss some of the drama as you're taken over by the familiarity of the tunes and you love them. It's also that the absolutely captivating thing that Verdi does even better than Puccini is that it is framed . . . you know when one piece ends and another begins. In Verdi's writing it's quite methodically organised. And if you are just listening and doing something else, or even if you are just sitting and contemplating, that organisation's great. It sort of organises your mind. I prefer it to the great swirls or drifts of sound like, for example, the music of Mahler. In that sense Verdi is much easier to listen to and much more compelling. Of course I've quite liked imposing order on my life so imposing order in music is a good thing too. For instance, Schoenberg and Berg might use a very different tonal system but it is very disciplined. A lot of music of today is just not disciplined.

MB: There's almost a kind of anti-discipline about it?

Baroness Neuberger: Yes, I think it's synthetic a lot of it and I think that's a real shame because it ought to work rather better. Music has got to have some intellectual content . . . some methodology. I may not share the methodology and I may not like it but at least I may begin to understand it. If your work is about divine inspiration . . . fine – but divine inspiration should encourage you to put some method into it. To me it's like some of this abstract stuff . . . it's just all over the place!

MB: If music was to be taken away from you what would that be like?

Baroness Neuberger: Terrible, absolutely terrible. I mean I think it's quite possible I might go deaf, many of us do in later life. At the moment I've got quite sharp hearing but at 55 that changes. At 55 you realise it's beginning to happen. My vision got worse but that's just ageing and one does it as gracefully as one can . . . but I think that going deaf would be terrible. And I wonder if one of the reasons my father didn't listen to music more was that he was becoming deaf. It was just too difficult. I realise that my father became deaf, my mother became a bit deaf and I think my chances are quite high . . . I think it would be terrible. But I suppose if you know enough music you can hear it in your head.

MB: That's true and a very important point isn't it? You can get a cue, a fragment of a piece of music, and carry it on in your head?

Baroness Neuberger: Yes . . . if I am on my own, driving somewhere and playing something in the car, I listen to quite a lot of choral music of one sort or another and I quite like being able to join in provided nobody's listening! (laughter).

MB: A sort of sing-along-with . . .

Baroness Neuberger: Yes I do . . . and I might well have Jessye Norman blasting . . . and I carry on and join in . . . which is quite funny. So I suppose if you go deaf you would be worried about joining in because you wouldn't know whether you were in tune or not. And I'm not good enough to feel it. Some people can feel the rhythm, the vibration . . . I can't.

MB: What do you listen *for*?

Baroness Neuberger: A mixture of things . . . relaxation, inspiration, intellectual stimulation and all sorts of other reasons . . . but I don't think I'm listening *out* for anything in particular.

MB: You don't have a preconception about . . . finding something in music?

Baroness Neuberger: No, I think music is a language . . . and one of the reasons that opera is so important to me is that it allows you to have the musical language and the words and the visual. So you have all the possible languages except for touch and that's why I think it is so powerful as a medium. It's all-embracing in a way that some music never manages. That's because of the quality of the music . . . although there are some fine examples of solo music, but they are very rare. I suppose I think it's also a language in which things are expressed that it's hard to express in words. But I don't think I'm listening *for* anything in particular. Music has a variety of affect and I know it is a very important part of my life.

There are lots of people who have huge collections of CDs, huge collections of books on music, but I'm not like that at all. It's very much a happy but not a professional part of my life.

MB: Mmn . . .

Baroness Neuberger: But it's extraordinarily important to me and one of the things that keeps me going. We had a Service of Passover yesterday and we were quite a large number and we were almost singing 'a cappella' and that was tremendously moving. We didn't have our normal choir, we just had our Cantor. There is one member of the congregation who is an absolutely brilliant singer and I am able to stay in tune, so there were three of us leading and we could sing everything in parts and that was just lovely . . . just with the congregation and that is very important to me . . . it's spiritually important. I think it is especially significant for me in a religious context. But I don't think that music is only spiritual.

MB: Exactly . . . John Sloboda the music psychologist writes very interestingly that some music is also about communion. . . . What might this be about?

Baroness Neuberger: I do think that you are able to hear things in music that you find difficult to express in words, that's clear. I think you can have a lyrical ecstasy that I never get from the spoken word . . . offer me the theatre and I say don't bother. I just don't get it. Whereas take me to the opera, and even if it's an opera I'm not particularly fond of there will be moments where I'm completely hooked, but 'communion'? . . . well I suppose 'communion' is a bit difficult if you are Jewish.

MB: But if we go back to the infant/mother relationship and the start of music?

Baroness Neuberger: No, I think it's different . . . no, I don't think that is quite right. If you have 'and all flesh is as grass' in the Brahms *Requiem* and I think that Brahms was a profoundly religious man . . . strong Protestant tradition, rather *Old Testament* in a funny kind of way . . . but which speaks to me very strongly. I think I have moments listening to that where I feel that if you had emotional heart strings they are pulled quite hard. And I think there is perhaps a spiritual sense of the relationship between the Divine which is eternal and human beings who are mortal. And music expresses that as much as the words and the words are themselves incredible . . . very fine, and in themselves very expressive. Is that spiritual communion? I'm not quite sure. That's the nearest I get. I think it's more about something else. I think it's about recognising an essential truth in the words and the music at the same time. It's plangent and I think that's the bit that's so powerful.

MB: Thank you Baroness Neuberger.

CHAPTER 4

Conversation with Benjamin Zephaniah

Benjamin Zephaniah is a poet, and this conversation took place in Birmingham City Library.

MB: What would you say, Benjamin, to introduce yourself to the reader?

Benjamin: My full name is Benjamin Obediah Ifrahim Zephaniah. I always say that makes me Christian, Moslem and Jewish. I do think of myself as a created being and some people say I'm a political writer, but I don't really understand politics. I write about the world around me, which obviously makes me write about politics or the results of politics and I'll use anything necessary to express myself. That's why you find me writin' plays, novels, music, dance pieces . . . whatever it takes to express that emotion, feelin', whatever it is, I'll use it. It's just a matter . . . for me . . . of tryin' to convey messages . . . tryin' to get people to think for themselves.

MB: This seems very important to you . . . getting people to think for themselves . . . you say that quite a lot in your writing.

Benjamin: That's the most important thing for me. People say 'Do you have a political line? Or are you trying to convert me to anything?'. No I don't. I don't expect people always to agree with me. But if they watch me perform on stage I want them to go away sayin', 'Well I might disagree with him here and there but at least he's got the guts to get up there and say what he feels and maybe I should do that sometimes in my life'. And that can be anythin' . It could be going away writin' to your MP or maybe it's sayin' to the man in your life that you're not going to stay tied to the kitchen or whatever.

MB: Or even that you're not going to stay with him?

Benjamin: Exactly . . . or whatever it is. Just have the confidence to express yourself.

MB: When did you come over to this country, Benjamin?

Benjamin: I was born here.

MB: Oh, you were born here . . . somehow I thought you were born in Jamaica and came over here.

Benjamin: No, I was born in this city not very far from where we sit right now. There are web sites that have me born in Jamaica or Yugoslavia . . . .

MB: But you went to Jamaica?

Benjamin: Yes, and I went there a lot to visit my grandparents. But you can hear this in my poetry and the way I speak . . . you can hear the influence of Jamaica.

MB: Yes, yes. It's very kind of you to take the time to have this conversation . . . everybody wants a bit of your time now . . . me included. But it hasn't always been like this for you . . . I'm thinking about you when you were 14 or 15?

Benjamin: Mmn . . .

MB: I wonder what life was like for you then?

Benjamin: It's interesting . . . it was the opposite. I wanted to talk to people . . . I remember being excluded from school and in those days being excluded from school wasn't like now where you have all those exclusion programmes. You were just left on the street. And . . . in my case my mother, who was trying to earn a livin' and my father, who was tryin' to earn a livin', were struggling to provide. So they weren't really able to take time off to look after me. So I was left on the street.

MB: So when was that, 19 . . .?

Benjamin: Early to mid-70s. Now I was excluded because I was an unruly boy and not paying attention in class really and I was tired at school. Now if they had spoken to me they would have realised that. Hey, you know he's tired at school; he's been up 'til three o'clock in the morning listenin' to his mother and father fightin' all night . . . you know, he's come to school without any breakfast and there's all this friction goin' on at home. When he left the house and walked down the street he was being stopped and searched by the police, so by the time he comes into school of course he's an angry young man . . . nobody listened.

MB: Yes.

Benjamin: Well nobody asked questions. It was assumed you were a bad boy and this is what's going to happen to you . . . so it was kind of lonely, which is why I've got this thing of speakin' my mind now. And gettin' people to listen, to not just me but to other people . . . I know it makes the world a better place if we try to 'overstand'.

MB: Could you say a bit more about 'overstand'?

Benjamin: Well you know it's a very Jamaican thing. We take English words that don't quite fit what we really want them to say and we change them . . . So, an oppressor becomes a 'downpressor' because they press you down. An official is a 'high official' because they are higher. A politician will say he understands you but he gets your vote and walks all over you. So you've been 'understood'. So we say 'overstood' which means more empathy with you.

MB: Right . . . there's more empathy with 'overstand'.

Benjamin: When you really connect with their suffering . . . or you really feel what they're goin' through . . . That's 'overstandin''. If you were a woman really in touch with the plight of another woman you would say, 'I know that' . . . that's 'overstandin''. I think it's because people over-use 'understand', so it loses its meaning. For example, people say 'I understand what's happenin' for the poor people in Iraq and, guess what now, I'm just goin' to get on with my dinner and get it out of my mind'. If you really understand what's happenin' to the people of Iraq you will know or identify with the story I heard the other day. A young boy went to the bathroom and brushed his teeth, sat down at the breakfast table and a bomb hit him. A friend of mine who was interviewin' him said, 'So what happened to you?,' and he said, 'I lost one leg but it's OK, the lad next door he died'. And you think, God, there's this young boy who thinks it's OK because he's got one leg.

MB: Yes, yes.

Benjamin: So you think about our situation, if you're a kid, you get up and clean your teeth . . . what can go wrong? You can forget your books or something like that . . . minor things. We don't wake up in Birmingham and think a bomb is going to explode . . . it's so removed from our day-to-day reality.

MB: It is.

Benjamin: And I remember . . . just to bring it back home a bit . . . without being party political. I remember goin' to Northern Ireland and going into Woolworths and British Home Stores and findin' troops at the door. And I thought this is only a few miles from Birmingham and I just couldn't imagine goin' into a shop in Birmingham with troops pointin' a gun at you as you walk in . . . and I thought do people in England and outside Northern Ireland really understand what it's like, and that's when I think we need to 'overstand'. It's difficult because we are so very far removed from that reality . . . but I think if you stretch your imagination . . . you can connect in some way. You're not goin' to get the full picture if you don't.

MB: Perhaps when you say 'understand' we're using only thinking . . . and with 'overstand' we're using feeling and thinking?

Benjamin: Yes, yes . . . you can logically understand but you really need to feel it too.

MB: What was the music you listened to most when you were 14 or 15?

Benjamin: Well . . . it was an interestin' mixture you know because the music that we played and the records we had were kind of 'ska' music which is a kind of reggae. This is the music that Bob Marley was associated with before it evolved into reggae. So it was early Jamaican popular music . . . but there was also the music of the Church.

MB: Yes . . . right.

Benjamin: What would be called Gospel Songs . . . but they didn't call it Gospel Songs . . . they called it Praise. They were happy clappy songs, *Praise ye the Lord* . . . very upliftin' songs sung in church . . . tambourines, drums. (At this point Benjamin gave a vocal demonstration accompanied by complex rhythms on the back of a chair and table.) And I remember lookin' at the English churches and thinkin' . . . they're so quiet! (some laughter and smiles). Do they really want to praise God? Cos the Bible says 'Praise Him loud', 'make a joyful noise unto God', 'praise him with the tambourine and drum and stuff ' . . . and the churches in England seemed so depressed. They should be happy if they're praisin' God. They're sayin' 'thank you for life, for all we have', but they just seem to be there because they're being told to. That's the impression we had when we went home and talked about it. We would turn on the television on Sunday and we would hear *Stand Up, Stand Up for Jesus* (sung in a mournful voice by Benjamin). Sometimes we would be singin' the same song but it would be *Stand Up, Stand Up for Jesus* (sung by Benjamin with a lively rhythmic accompaniment on the back of the chair).

MB: When you sing that, you move with it. I think that music for you must be about movement?

Benjamin: It's physical. It's not just something that happens with the throat and the mouth. Singin' for us happens with the hands and the feet . . . everything. And then alongside that I listened to every kind of swing music I suppose . . . Paul Anka and even people like Frank Sinatra. That's the kind of thing I listened to on the radio. I listened to them on a little transistor. I have always listened to all kinds of music from 'rock' to 'reggae' or 'ska'. I've never been one of those people who says, 'This is *my* music', excluding other kinds of music.

MB: What did music mean for you then?

Benjamin: Well . . . it meant many things . . . . There were two stages in my life. There was one where I was kind of catchin' on to my mother's dress and I listened to what my mother listened to, which was Gospel music, Frank Sinatra, early ska . . . and then it meant praisin' God. It meant we used to sing so much that people in the congregation started 'speakin' in tongues' and going into what people would think of as a kind of fit, they got so taken over by the Holy Spirit. So it was quite dramatic to watch. Bodies would fall on the floor gyratin' . They would fly through the air because they're taken over by the Holy Spirit. And all of this is induced by the singin' and the drums. Then there were also family 'get-togethers' where there were community songs . . . lots of Jamaican songs about markets. So these songs made us a community. These were Jamaican songs that no-one else sang.

MB: Yes, yes.

Benjamin: Then there were the Frank Sinatra songs . . . these were the outside world. The other stage is when I move away from my mother and start pickin' my own music and thinkin' for myself.

MB: How old were you then?

Benjamin: I would say 14 . . . and when I started to do that I started picking the music of Bob Marley and Peter Tosh . . . Peter Mackintosh really. And at this point I started to get involved with the Rastafarian movement. Now one can think of Rastafarians as a branch of Christianity in a way. As Rastafarians we always are writing the Third Testament – a continuation of Christianity, so we look at the *Bible* and we recognise the *Bible* but we have a very black spin on it.

MB: Right.

Benjamin: We don't paint Jesus as this blue-eyed, blond-haired man.

MB: I don't think he did have blue eyes and blond hair.

Benjamin: No, his family came out of Egypt and slavery and He was born in Palestine and maybe by all descriptions he was a black man with dreadlocks like me! Anyway He had long hair and you read in the *Bible* of Solomon who says 'I am black but I am, comely' and he talks about his locks. So it was lookin' at the Bible through black spectacles and usin' it as a kind of Liberation Theology and that we wanted to go to heaven like other religious people, go to paradise. *But* . . . we also wanted freedom on earth! So when you hear Bob Marley, 'Get up, stand up, stand up for your rights', if you listen to the words very carefully he says 'We're sick and tired of this hissin', kissin' game – dyin' to go to heaven in Jesus' name.'

MB: Yes . . . .

Benjamin: 'For we know and we understand Almighty God is a livin' man. You can fool some people sometimes but you can't fool all the people all the time. And now we've seen the light, we get to stand up for our rights . . .', and then he says 'Most people think great God will come here from the sky, take away everything and make everyone feel high. But you know what life is worth, you will look for yours on earth, and now you see the light you stand up for your right!'

MB: This is really very Christian.

Benjamin: Yes . . . in fact they say that Marx wouldn't be a Marxist and Christ wouldn't be a Christian today! The only record we have of Christ goin' into a church he smashed it up! He'd say what's all this capitalism goin' on in here; all this wheelin' and dealin'.

MB: All this money!

Benjamin: Yeah . . . and what did he do? He spent all his time on the street with lepers. And he was very sympathetic with the women. You know someone who was reputed to be a prostitute touched his feet.

MB: Mary Magdalene.

Benjamin: Yeah, so if Christ were alive today he'd be with the AIDS patients. He would probably be walkin' around the 'red light' district talkin' to the women. And he wouldn't be spendin' all his time in Church.

MB: Yes, kneeling.

Benjamin: Yeah . . . it's ironic. It was a kind of liberation therapy of music. It was connected to spirituality and political consciousness. That's what it meant to me then.

MB: There's an oral tradition, Benjamin, of performing poetry in your culture. I was going to say in your first culture, but that's not quite right now. Do you have a first culture and a second culture?

Benjamin: You see . . . growin' up in Handsworth it *was* like growin' up in Jamaica at that time. We spoke Jamaican . . . I know that Jamaicans speak English of course. But they have a particular take on the language. But we ate Jamaican, all the neighbours were Jamaican. I remember when I was very young my mother told me that an uncle was comin' from Jamaica. So I went to Handsworth park and stood on the highest point to catch him comin' up the hill because I thought that Jamaica was just on the outskirts of Birmingham (much laughter).

MB: That's lovely.

Benjamin: Everything was very, very Jamaican. We lived in . . . Jamaican space . . . a bit like a Jamaican embassy. It was a bit of Jamaican culture in Britain . . . I called Handsworth the English capital of Jamaica . . . In this country, in western old-fashioned culture when mother wanted to teach a girl a recipe, you would take her to the kitchen and say 'You add some salt and mix etc.'. When my mother did this she did it in rhyme . . .

MB: Ah . . .

Benjamin: There were of course practical instructions but you would have the poem first. (Benjamin then demonstrated in rhythmic verse.) You take a bit of this . . . You take a bit of that . . . You add a bit of this . . . You add a bit of that . . . .

MB: So your mother spoke to you in rhyme.

Benjamin: Yes, yes. I remember . . . but because of tradition the boys didn't cook so my mother tried to teach me the months of the year (to a beat) . . . 30 days September, April, June and November . . . all the rest are 31 except . . . . It was always like that and because we were illiterate everything was remembered by rhyme. The women who came over in those days were not highly educated. My mother was a country girl . . . not completely illiterate but not the best reader in the world so she compensated by using the old tradition of rhythm and rhyme to remember things. It wasn't art . . . it was a very functional process.

MB: Would you say it was folk art?

Benjamin: Yes, it was folk art but my mother would say she was just bein' practical.

MB: In your CD *Naked* . . ., which is poetry with music . . . you write in the second poem that God will liberate those who liberate themselves. Was there any one person who saw your exceptional talent and helped you to liberate yourself?

Benjamin: I have to be *really* honest and say 'No'. I'll tell you why that is . . . because even though my mum recognised my talent she said 'Son' (in them days you know), 'Get an apprenticeship. Come on . . . forget this literature and poetry and stuff. It's good around the house. It's an important part of our culture . . . but you're never goin' to earn a livin' from it. You'll starve. This is a white man's country.' I remember she said to me one day 'You tell me, you name me, one white man that you know who's earnin' a livin' from this?'

MB: (Laughter).

Benjamin: Mmm . . . William Shakespeare . . . and she said 'Him dead a long time ago. If a white man can't earn a livin' this way how can you as a young black man livin' in the ghetto.'

MB: She had a point.

Benjamin: Yea, I thought she was being very protective. People said it was good what you were doin' but don't think of it very seriously . . . and I tell you what I did. When I was about 15 or so I wrote a letter to Bob Marley and I sent him some poems . . . and he wrote back. Now this is why any child . . . anyone . . . who writes a letter to me gets a reply. Because when I read his letter he said, 'Keep it up, you're doin' good work. I'm very inspired.' . . . .Oh, Bob Marley inspired by my work . . . and he's tellin' me that it's good and I should keep it up. So in a way the answer to your question is 'yes' . . . and it came from Bob Marley.

MB: And your story earlier when you were 14 reminds me of your book *Gangsta Rap* and the man in that book in charge of the music shop, Marga Man. So maybe Bob Marley was your Marga Man.

Benjamin: Yeah, although he wasn't with me.

MB: But he 'saw' you, he 'recognised' you.

Benjamin: Yes, yes it does help if you've got someone to say 'Keep it up, you're doin' well' because if you're writing . . . creatin' poetry in my mind all the time . . . it can be a very lonely world you know. Now-a-days most librarians have outreach programmes, writin' groups and you can practise writin', share writin'. They have connections with local publishers. In my days there was nothin'.

MB: How did you get out of this?

Benjamin: Well what happened was that I started creating poetry. My mother was right in one sense that you had to be realistic and earn a livin'. And because of racism and high unemployment in those days I got involved in crime and I went to an approved school and borstal. And all the time I was walkin' around sayin' 'But I'm a poet. I shouldn't be here'. But when I came out (I was livin' in Northfield, a part of Birmingham) hand guns had just started to come on to the street . . . up until then it had been mainly shotguns, and you had to be really well-connected to get a shotgun. But suddenly hand guns were available very cheaply. And I started to see my friends being shot or gettin' arrested and gettin' very long sentences, not 18 months like me . . . more 10–15 years, and I thought by the law of averages I'll be somewhere next along the line. So I woke up one day and said 'I'm getting out of here'. So I went to London. Not that London was any better and in many ways London was more dangerous. But . . . I was a blank canvas so I could mix with a different crowd of people.

MB: Yes, yes.

Benjamin: And immediately I started mixin' with other kinds of reggae musicians and the punk musicians of the time. And the 'alternative cabaret' before they were famous . . . Alexei Sayle, Ben Elton, French and Saunders . . . and that's when I started performin'. That's when I got picked up by the mainstream.

MB: That's a great story and great that you did it!

Benjamin: I went to the East End of London and I tried to get published with a normal publisher. Some of them would just look at me . . . and I don't blame them, I think it was a lack of overstanding! They would say 'Oh we don't do black Rastafarian poetry you know'. Anyone who looks at me will know that I'm a black Rastafarian but in a culture novels reach everyone. But most of my books do not sell to black people. They sell to everyone. If I did manage to sell to every black person in Britain, I'd just about earn a livin'. If you're professional you've got to broaden out.

MB: So . . . would that include your performances?

Benjamin: The publishers rejected me so then I started performin' . . . and then there was a small collective that decided to publish a book of mine which did alright. Then somebody asked me to perform at North East London Polytechnic. I performed there and I did it free and he said would I come back next week. After that show he gave me £5, and the next week £10. After the third week it was £15 . . . but there was a man in the audience called Roland Muldoon who is now the director of the Hackney Empire, London. He came to me and said 'You know when comedians go on stage and start with a joke about a black man, an Irish man and an English man, or they go on stage with mother-in-law jokes . . . well I'm promotin' poets, musicians, and comedians that *don't* do that. It's called 'alternative cabaret' and I've got somebody called Dawn French and Ben Elton and we're doin' tours around the country and we'd like you to come and join us.'

MB: Great!

Benjamin: And I said 'OK'. I didn't really understand all of what it was about but I understood the principle non-racist, non-sexist and that was me. I started doing that and then Channel 4 started and in those days Channel 4 was an 'alternative'. It was a place where women and black people had a voice. And back in those days in the 1980s we were all wantin' a voice.

MB: Now you write in *Dis is Me Naked* . . . 'Dis is my music, loud, deep jungle music.' Could you say a bit more about that, Benjamin?

Benjamin: Well . . . in this poem, I'm really tryin' to be as honest as I can. I'm tryin' to bring my personal and political thoughts and feelin's together. When I say 'Dis is my music', heavy, loud music . . . this is the music where I feel at home. This is me expressin' myself. It goes on to say 'We made this music, we made love and riots to this music'. We created this magic but we still don't own this magic . . . it's owned by the record companies.

MB: Yes, yes.

Benjamin: 'How long will we struggle for our royalty cheque?' I really do believe we are creative bein's and this music comes from the street. Then it gets gobbled up by the record companies and they give us a small percentage of it and take away our rights to own it, and we feel grateful because we get a little bit of a percentage. It's about this kind of *ownership* of the music. It's also partly about lookin' at me naked, personally and emotionally naked. I need this music to express myself, express my feelin's here. Sometimes it's loud, sometimes the language is a bit raw. I swear! . . . this is how I feel . . . this is me . . . this is really me.

MB: Now . . . How would you describe the effect of the music in poem number 4: *When I See You I Know Life Was Made for Livin'*? This is a very different kind of music.

Benjamin: In this song, it's the closest thing I've got to a love song with a woman. So, I'm in the room with my lover and I say 'When I see you I know life was made for livin, when I see you I want to make love to you physically. I think goin' to bed with you is great, I want to touch your body but *first* I want to touch your mind.' It's really easy to have sexual intercourse . . . kids do it behind the bicycle shed. But to have mental intercourse . . . is a very different thing. So you see young people now 'I like her man, she moves nice man', but as soon as there is some little difficulty in the relationship, it all falls apart. They don't really know how each other feels. And that's what the poem is about. It's about trying to understand or overstand each other.

MB: It has a lovely swing to it. To me it's like an adult lullaby . . . I don't know if that makes sense to you?

Benjamin: That makes sense . . . it's like another poem, I'm very proud of. It's a poem about my mum, *I Love My Mother and My Mother Loves Me*. These are poems that men find very difficult to like. It tends to be all 'rock and roll baby'. Men find it very easy to write about sex and dancin' and about being tough, but if it's about wantin' to connect with a woman intellectually . . . a lot of men find that very difficult.

MB: Benjamin, you've written a lot of poetry without musical accompaniment and some poems like *Dis is Me Naked* appear with and without music. Now, does it feel different for you with a musical accompaniment?

Benjamin: Yes . . . I have to wait for the music . . . well, I think musically and I think the words. When I perform a poem without music I think the spoken words have to make a kind of music. I remember one of my big ambitions was to be able to stand on stage and perform a poem and watch people dance to the poem without music. And I remember at one of my performances somebody did it!

MB: Oh, great!

Benjamin: Sometimes a poem flows with the rhythm and you don't need music. But when I use music in a performance I have to *wait* for it. I'm the kind of poet that has to slow down to the music. Other poets have to speed up. Sometimes I will write a poem and hear a piece of music which will go with it and which will work. When I perform my poetry to music it makes people go and buy the book. I like to bring literature into the dance hall. When I'm workin' with musicians, though, I say to them it's not the case of you makin' music and I'm goin' to shout over you. Now here are the words and I want you to wrap the music around them. The musicians have to realise that some people in the audience will know the words, so let them hear them. Don't get in the way of the words. The job of the musician is to enhance the poem. Don't play too loud, don't play over me.

MB: It has been said that music shares a sense of passing time. Does this have a meaning for you when you choose poetry and music together?

Benjamin: Passing time . . . it's interestin' that . . . *Gangsta Rap* has been turned into a musical for the Theatre Royal in London. And when we were workin' with the director he kept talkin' about music and how it makes the time pass . . . so in the novel I may have three chapters but in the musical we can't speak word for word these three chapters, so we have a song which over a short space of time describes what is in these three chapters . . .

MB: And it *takes* time to do this.

Benjamin: In another sense you lose track of time. You're workin' with time because music's about time but you go into a funny place. When you're soundin' that note or sayin' those words that's all there is in the world . . . .

MB: It's like another level.

Benjamin: This makes me think of cosmology and the whole concept of time and in one of my poems I say, 'Time is somethin' that stops everythin' happenin' at once'.

MB: It gives you a space to live.

Benjamin: With the language we have, it's a real struggle to break it down to a sentence or so. And one of the depressin' things about modern-day music, popular music, is that what is created must be brought down to 3½ minutes by the radio stations. So when record companies are sayin' no music more than 4 minutes because the radio stations won't play it and people won't hear it . . . that's the sad thing. If I'm asked how long is my poem or my piece of music I will answer, 'As long as it takes'. The great poets like Shelley and Keats and composers like Beethoven and Mozart. They had time and weren't bombarded with record companies, they had time to think of the people in front of them. And however long the piece took, they took that long. And that's so beautiful because it means that you, the audience, when you come to listen to the poem or the piece of music you must invest in it. You're not thinkin' 3½ minutes. 'Impress me in 3½ minutes!'

MB: On investing in time. Is there something about time passing horizontally as it were in your poetry? Is your sense of time different now that you are 47 from when you were 37?

Benjamin: I think I used to take time for granted. I know that when I was 27, makin' a record was just makin' the next record. I remember I got very depressed on my 30th birthday because do this again and I'm 60. But I tell you now, if I'm goin' to invest time in creatin' this piece of music or poetry I won't waste it. Don't waste it because as you get older you are more aware that you can leave earth at any time through natural causes or un-natural causes. When you're young you feel invincible. So I don't want time to pass . . . I don't want to look back and say I wasted time. But I don't think I have. I think my big weakness is that I'm probably too obsessed with time and my work and don't give enough time to my family. I don't have children but my mother tells me I spend all my time workin' and 'Why don't you sit down for an hour?'

There's somethin' I always wanted to do and I've now done it. It's when you drive up to a place and look at the house and say to your mum, 'Mum do you like that?' and she says, 'Yes' and I buy it and say, 'Mum it's yours'.

MB: That's really lovely.

Benjamin: And then I put her in it . . . then run away . . . and just pop in now and again and she says, 'When are you goin' to come and stay?'

MB: It's really hard this.

Benjamin: I'm so obsessed with working and making sure I get this done and that done on time.

MB: As I said at the beginnin' everybody wants a bit of you now . . . music, rhythm and movement are so much part of you, Benjamin, if this was taken away from you can you imagine what that would be like?

Benjamin: Oh gosh . . . no . . . if you took away all the physical means. If you stopped me goin' to the recording studios and readin' poetry I would still use the body as an instrument. The people who wanted to be with me durin' the day would still want me . . . (At this point Benjamin tapped out a complicated rhythm with his fingers on the back of the chair) . . . I've got the beat goin' now (as he elaborated the rhythm with syncopation).

MB: You've got your percussion going there . . . .

Benjamin: I use everything as an instrument . . . I've still got my body and if I can't do that I'll still make music in my head. I just think human bein's need music . . . every culture has music. I've met people who don't like one kind of music or another. But I've never met anyone who doesn't like music at all . . . There's always something. It could be the most simple music or the most complicated. When I don't like some music I just say 'It's not for me. It's not my thing'. Most music is OK in fact. If people like loud crashin' heavy metal music I will try and understand it and try and find out what is in it for that group of people.

  I went to a concert last night with a band called the Kaiser Chiefs and I'm pretty sure I was the oldest person there. I was right down in the middle of the dance floor . . . and they don't dance now, they just jump up and down. And you've a struggle to stay on your feet but I soon got into it. And I looked back and there were all these hundreds of people and not a black face. And it made me think . . . perhaps black people tend to like the bass, the reggae, the funk, the blues and the rhythm . . . but it was a very enjoyable night. It helped me understand these young people and the way they sing along is a bit like football chantin'. When I hear parents say I don't understand the music my kids listen to, I say you've got to try and understand it because then you are really trying to connect with your kids.

MB: You're about to present a TV programme on slavery quite soon, Benjamin. Would you agree that you are a fine example of a truly liberated human being?

Benjamin: There's an old Bob Marley song which says 'Emancipate yourself from mental slavery – none but ourselves can free our mind'. What he's sayin' is that it's one thing to get free of your chains and shackles and physical slavery, but to emancipate ourselves from mental slavery, that's for us to do personally. And it's not about the black man being oppressed or anything. You the white woman can also be in mental slavery. And so I think as far as that is concerned I am liberated. I'm very free thinkin'. Once upon a time I would go with the crowd and I think that's a kind of slavery. I remember when I was a kid I used to go out beatin' up gays – I don't do that now. The idea of just followin' the crowd . . . I feel so confident in myself I don't feel the need to go with the crowd. I always say that the most important thing you can do is to think for yourself. If you don't you can get to believe that black kids are always on the margins or black kids don't care about British justice. You've got to learn to think for yourself. I don't think that religion was part of God's plan. It can give God a bad name!

MB: Thank you very much Benjamin.

CHAPTER 5

A gathering of musical experiences

In Chapters 1–4 we have been privileged to hear what music has meant for four people in the public eye. They have not all been trained in the discipline of music to the level of Professor Mercedes Pavlicevic, but they each have an abundance of communicative musicality.

Communicative musicality, which we will consider in more detail later, is, according to Stephen Malloch, 'The art of human companionable communication . . .. It is the vehicle which carries emotion from one to another and it is our ability to move sympathetically with one another.'[1]

We notice it most clearly in healthy normal infant–mother communication or any companionable communication with a baby, no matter how young. If all goes reasonably well with our development as babies and we do not experience severe trauma, which might derail our reaching out to others, this capacity to engage non-verbally with another is with us for life. Being in lively verbal communication with another as adults could also be called communicative musicality, but it is the non-verbal ways of being with another person that interest us here and especially in psychotherapy, which traditionally has been regarded as 'the talking cure'. This however would be emphasising the verbal aspect of psychotherapy. The experience of listening to music chosen by the patient in the consulting room is the main subject of enquiry in this book and it is more than a talking cure and this will be discussed more fully later. But returning to the conversations in the last four chapters, none of the interviewees were patients of mine in any sense and each was asked what music meant for them. So what might we learn from these conversations about the experience of listening to music?

Each responded in some depth and recalled moments of listening to music in their lives which had been made more meaningful because of it. Mercedes Pavlicevic recalled the playing of Yo Yo Ma and the Chilean group Inti-Illimani where their playing was such that she experienced the music as being at one with it: 'I listen and become it with my entire being, not just my mind'. For Baroness Neuberger, when the essential truth of the words and music come together as in the Brahms *Requiem*, it perhaps captures for her the relationship between the eternal divine and the mortal human being. Music is so important for Katie Melua that she thinks of it sometimes as the sound track of life.

Benjamin Zephaniah's life is that of someone who lives rhythm and movement. He lives and communicates naturally through music, non-verbal sounds and rhythms and he is someone who is also a poet who captures words with his musical artistry. He writes that 'Human beings need music'.

Music is so much a part of each of their lives that not one can imagine a life without it. But what more can be said about music? We will now consider these experiences more closely to find different ways in which music can be understood.

What music is

Benjamin Zephaniah and Mercedes Pavlicevic experienced music as movement and energy as motion. Benjamin writes of being brought up in rhythm, and Mercedes describes how she becomes the energy in music which 'flows her'. Here they are both describing what music is for them, their personal philosophy of music. Both of these points of view start with the encounter of music 'out there' as it were. This objective view of music would seem to resonate with the philosophy of Zuckerkandl who writes that 'music is motion in the dynamic field of tones'.[2] This is not to say that they only experience music as 'out there' but it is the particular lens through which they viewed music at the time of the conversation. As Mercedes says, 'Music is always in context'. When Mercedes and Benjamin described their experience of music they were at that time describing this dynamic field of tones.

Katie Melua's and Baroness Neuberger's basic positions seem to resonate more particularly with the personal relational experience of music. They connect with music as symbolic of interpersonal relationships. Again this does not mean that they only view music in this way, they also experience music objectively. It is just a matter of emphasis, and of context.

Katie writes of a *Far Away Voice* in memory of Eva Cassidy and Baroness Neuberger's recollection of *Dido and Aeneas* is associated with the death of her father. These are intensely interpersonal musical experiences. Susanne Langer is the philosopher who held the view that music was a symbol of the structure of our inner emotional lives.[3] For Langer, music was more to do with our experiences as persons-in-relationship than it was to do with music as a phenomenon 'out there' in the world. These different philosophical views will be discussed more fully in the next chapter.

The group experience

A second way in which the four interviewees talked about music is the experience of listening to music in a group or groups. Here we would be discussing the experience of music from a sociological perspective rather than an individual one. Mercedes writes of the experience of being in a group as a child singing at St Peter's in Rome. She remembers the excitement, the performance, the fasting and being hungry, how time was slow. Then there was the competitiveness with the other choir, and then being caught up in the collective passion of the event with the arrival of the Pope. She also recalls being at a folk festival in Edinburgh and being aware of the different energies within the audience in the room and how music could 'collect people', focus this energy perhaps. This notion of how musical energy collects people is touched on in the next chapter when music at the Olympic Games is discussed.

Benjamin writes about the Jamaican Community in Birmingham and how music binds this group. He writes that there were a lot of Jamaican songs about markets, which were narratives of Jamaican life. Gospel songs were also very important in forging and supporting group identity. De Nora writes about music as a resource we turn to in the 'care of self' in a sociological context and this will be considered in the next chapter.[4]

Playing music in the school orchestra is a memory of group music-making for Baroness Neuberger and also singing in the West London Synagogue choir. When we talked about listening to music within a hospital context, we explored the difficulties of playing music in a public place and how the music chosen would not be to everyone's taste. We agreed that this whole area was sensitive and a solution was difficult. Perhaps one answer would be to have no music in public areas and a sitting room where a choice of music *would* be available. Other forms of 'art in movement', where changing scenes are projected on to a wall with natural sounds such as bird song and the sound of the wind in the trees, are creative ideas in some hospitals.

Katie Melua's early memory of a Georgian male voice choir made a deep impression on her, as did the folk music of Ireland and India. The tension between Catholic and Protestant groups in Northern Ireland underpinned her writing of the song *Belfast*, where she tried to capture the daily life of the people of Belfast as she saw it, and the tragedy of the situation. Here she was looking in on a group experience.

Everyday music and special music

Listening to the choices of music of the four interviewees, we could divide their experiences of music into the 'everyday' and the 'special'. The 'everyday' was the music they chose as background sound to other tasks and the 'special' seemed to have particular emotional significance for them.

Baroness Neuberger felt that the 'everyday' music 'gathered her concentration' when she was writing something lengthy, such as a chapter of a book. It was always classical and it could be the Brahms *Requiem* or Italian opera. It had to be familiar so that she could relax into it. The music though that is special to her is that which she really needs to attend to intellectually and emotionally, such as Bach, Handel or Purcell. One piece of music which was and is very special for her is *Dido and Aeneas*, which she played 'endlessly' when her father was dying.

'Everyday' music for Benjamin was and is Jamaican popular music such as 'reggae' and 'ska'. This was all around him while he was growing up, along with the Gospel songs from church. As he grew up he moved on to listening to Frank Sinatra songs and the music of Bob Marley and Peter Tosh. He writes that music that is 'special' to him is that which the composer has taken time over, and words and music together are very important for him. He writes that his music is 'loud deep jungle music' and he feels at home in this music, but he has also written a very lyrical love song *When I See You I Know that Life was Made for Livin'*, so we see two sides of 'special' music for Benjamin.

Working in the world of pop music, Katie is surrounded by music all the time. It is part of her profession to listen to what is being written and performed each day. In a sense this is her 'everyday' music, but she is aware that there are particular songs and artists who stand out, like the Beatles or Ella Fitzgerald. One singer in particular, Eva Cassidy, was very 'special' for Katie. Katie could recognise the particular beauty of her voice and her particular creative interpretation of the song *Somewhere over the Rainbow*. She was aware that Eva Cassidy stood out from the 'everyday' because she had the ability to reach her listeners very powerfully, to communicate with them authentically. Another instance of this ability of Katie to recognise the 'special' in pop music was her choice of Mike Batt's song *The Closest Thing to Crazy*. Not only does she hear that it is a good song, she also understands why. It is well constructed, as Benjamin has said above; it has taken time to write and someone has taken pains over it. Again, it is absolutely authentic emotionally.

We are now coming very near to committing the post-modern crime of saying that one piece of music may have more intrinsic value than another, and I will consider this in a moment. But first we will turn to the musical experiences of Mercedes.

Because Mercedes is so steeped in musical experiences, as her work involves improvising and listening to it, it was very difficult to find her 'everyday' music. In terms of music that she would engage in every day, her improvisation with patients would come first. But, she now does less of this as she is involved in training programmes and listening to music from all over the world to alert her students to the different genres and ways of playing. The 'everyday' and the 'special' categories of the experience of listening to music become unclear and blurred when she writes that her mood helps her choose the music that she listens to by choice. This would be a different perspective from notions of music as 'everyday' or 'special'. Mercedes' view is more individual, experiential and person-based, rather than considering what *music* is in relation to persons generally.

Mercedes writes that she 'will choose music that reflects her mood or amplifies it, or shifts it'. Her emphasis is on her *choice* and this by definition side-steps anything that is badly constructed or emotionally inadequate. It is unthinkable that she would willingly listen to music of poor quality or music which is mentally intrusive. She notes, however, that loud intrusive rock music coming from public loud-speakers in an underground station in Brussels was unacceptable. This is completely congruent with what she writes about choice and mood.

By choice, Mercedes listens to music that is 'expressive and not just chuntering along'. She needs music that breathes and enables her to breathe too. Her listening is very catholic in that she draws her choices from a very wide palette of musical genres, that is, from 'world music', along with classical music such as Bach, Brahms, Prokofiev and Shostakovich. She includes the African music of Youssou N'dour and the music from the Portuguese African colonies. The music of Sting, Simon and Garfunkel and sometimes Abba are noted along with the music of the Beatles, Eric Clapton, kd lang, Nusrat Ali Khan and many others.

But returning to the notion that one piece of music might have more value than another, Dissanayake takes up the challenge and argues that 'Ideas of beauty, quality and routes to transcendence do vary among human cultures and have to be learned. They are contingent and self-interested'.[5] She goes on to write that people in all societies have ideas of the beautiful and what is especially fine and they do make distinctions and note quality just as our four interviewees have done. In Benjamin's case, Bob Marley's music comes to mind; for Baroness Neuberger it would be Purcell's *Dido and Aeneas*; Katie's experience of listening to *Danny Boy* had particular meaning for her and Mercedes has listed many instances of musical experiences that were especially fine.

But Dissanayake holds the view that in a 'naturalistic aesthetics' such as she offers for consideration, learned criteria and learned responses, whether they are in the context of an African celebration or a Western symphonic concert of Mozart's music rest upon 'evolved universal propensities'.[5] But one might ask how these propensities evolve? Her response is that they begin in sensation,[6] which in human developmental terms means that they belong very early in our existence. In an earlier chapter, she writes of the young infant in response to a caretaker's loving attention:

> 'Instilled as part of our biological nature, the rhythms and modes of infancy demonstrate and develop the psychological capacities that predispose humans to mutuality the sharing of emotional states in patterned sequences with others. In the close early interactions between infants and their caretakers are the prototypes for what will become our later experiences of love, allegiance, art and other forms of self–transcendence.'[7]

Having established the origins of a 'naturalistic aesthetics', she describes four successive criteria for assigning aesthetic quality or 'aesthetic success' to an event such as a musical performance.[8] One piece of music each, already chosen by the interviewees from music that is in some way 'special', will be tested against the Dissanayake criteria for aesthetic quality. It will be noted how different this is from Mercedes' very personal and singular experiential perspective. Although she has a different philosophical view and doesn't enter into the discussion on aesthetic quality, there are areas of overlap, as will be seen.

Dissanayake's four criteria of aesthetic quality in her natural aesthetics are as follows.

Accessibility coupled with strikingness

Here Dissanayake describes the effect of a piece of music on our senses and thought and how we hear the rhythms, pitch and intervals that go to make up a piece of music. These must not only reach our senses, they must be notable. Katie's description of her experience of hearing *Danny Boy* would meet this first criterion. She writes of the 'bending of the note' for example. The music is accessible in that she is familiar with Irish melodies, and it is striking in the particular melodic nuance of the 'bending of the note'. The singing of Bob Marley had a striking impact on Benjamin as a young man. Bob Marley's music was accessible in that it had an authentic Jamaican rhythmic flow and Benjamin understood the powerful message in the words. It also gave him hope that *he* could be true to himself. The music of Purcell, especially *Dido and Aeneas*, combines accessibility and strikingness for Baroness Neuberger. She had been brought up in the 'habitus' of classical music, so listening to Purcell combined music that gripped the intellect with the beauty of sound for her. For Mercedes there are many pieces of music which fulfil this first criterion *depending on her mood*. In particular she selects the playing of Bach by Yo Yo Ma and the music of Inti-Illimani, the Chilean group of musicians. One of the reasons these pieces are accessible is because she is highly trained in music but they are also striking because of the 'exquisite ultra-sensitivity and virtuosity' of the playing, along with the beauty of sound and emotional communication.

Tangible relevance

This is the second criterion for a good or successful work. Along with being accessible and striking it will in addition have a tangible context in the particular life of the listener. In other words, it will have particular culturally embedded meaning for them in some way. Dissanayake quotes Nilotic Sudanese songs that 'evoke brilliant things about the central subject of that culture: cattle'. She continues, 'Without appreciating a work's tangible relevance to the cultural tradition in which it exists, we cannot expect to experience fully its emotional power'. Katie's awareness of Irish culture when she experiences the singing of *Danny Boy* would fulfil this criterion. Benjamin's choice of Bob Marley's music and its relevance to Jamaican culture fits this second criterion also. Mercedes' wide knowledge of the music of world cultures and the best examples of particularly striking music also meet this category of tangible relevance, as does Baroness Neuberger's choice of *Dido and Aeneas* with her understanding of the cultural text and the particular meaning and relevance it had when her father was dying.

Evocative resonance

Here, Dissanayake describes a complexity or density of meaning embodied in the work, in *addition* to the tangible cultural or individual interests. She writes that there will be 'more than meets the eye' in the complexity or density of meaning embodied in the work. Baroness Neuberger's choice of *Dido and Aeneas* would be an example of this third criterion. Here Baroness Neuberger links the story of *Dido and Aeneas* to the meetings with her father before he died. This music had an added personal sorrow attached to it which she remembers and which it evokes when she hears it. Katie's choice of *Danny Boy* is associated with the nostalgia of the stories of people who have left Ireland and the still warm memories of them by the groups of family, friends and neighbours left behind. This is so really meaningful for the people of Ireland who travelled worldwide to have a better life and were so missed by the people who were left behind. These kinds of feelings may be particularly evoked for Katie because she herself has travelled across the world as a child and has also left warm relationships behind. For Benjamin, listening to the songs of Bob Marley had extra evocative resonance for him because he became involved with the Rastafarian movement and his sense of identity as a black person was acknowledged and celebrated through Bob Marley's songs.

Satisfying fullness

This is the last and highest of the levels of perceived aesthetic value in a created composition for Dissanayake. Here, she writes that the listener or 'respondent' feels as if something has been accomplished by the work or activity, and a sense of completeness or sufficiency is felt. She continues that not every aesthetic experience is so complete, and such an experience may occur only once or twice in a lifetime, but when the three other characteristics – accessibility with strikingness, tangible relevance, and evocative resonance – are present, a high degree of fulfilment is usually felt and this is more common. This would still be a different experience from 'everyday' music. She writes:

> 'Such fulfilments arise when life interests are touched, experiential depths are sounded, greater possibilities are evoked, and the works that embody these have been constructed and composed with care and commitment but, I daresay, not otherwise.'[9]

Although we have not explored the sublime experience in particular, Mercedes' writing on recalling the playing of Yo Yo Ma and the Chilean group Inti-Illimani could be said to come near to this satisfying fullness perhaps. She writes, 'When I listen to artists like this then the music and I become one; I lose sense of the day, or time or place and become this energy which flows me, in a way, and allows me to allow it to flow me'. When Katie heard Eva Cassidy sing *Over the Rainbow*, she remembers exactly where she was. She writes, 'Suddenly this voice came on. There was just something about the voice – a cry of emotion – and her voice was crystal clear. Almost angelic.' This was also a memorable and powerful aesthetic experience for Katie. Baroness Neuberger writes that the Brahms *Requiem* speaks to her very strongly and she feels that if she had emotional heart strings, they would be pulled quite hard. At these times she writes, 'I think there is perhaps a spiritual sense of the relationship between the divine which is eternal and human beings who are mortal.' This would be a powerful aesthetic response to the Brahms *Requiem*. Benjamin's experience of Bob Marley singing *Get Up, Stand Up, Stand Up For Your Rights* was a very powerful aesthetic moment for him. This along with the Rastafarian movement was, as he says, 'a kind of Liberation Theology'. Rhythm, music and poetry are his natural aesthetic way of being in the world.

What have we learned about the experience of listening to music?

Drawing together what we have learned about the experiences of our four interviewees, it could now be said that music is embedded in the culture we have been brought up in. We may go on to find our 'own' music, but this will depend on the life experiences of the individual person. Within each group or culture there will be music that is considered among the best of that particular genre. From the simple to the complex, there will be those examples that the composer has taken pains over and it will be taken seriously by the composer and listeners. These examples will be recognised and experienced by the group or individual as having particular beauty, energy or emotional import. These compositions will be considered as 'special'.

'Everyday' music will be just that. It will not have any particular claim to being especially beautiful, striking or emotionally powerful or meaningful. It may be crafted just for fun and ease of listening. Dissanayake takes an interesting view on the values associated with such music. She writes that traditionally an artist or musician, when creating and elaborating a work of art to do with important life concerns, took time and care about it. She continues that in order to have beauty and quality in our lives we too must care about what we look at or listen to and that there are particular problems in the 21st century to do with the avenues through which we encounter art in all its forms. She writes:

> 'The "values" that suffuse our lives are additionally affected by the fact that the primary avenues for elaboration – advertisements and popular entertainment – have to compete among themselves for our attention. Because their ultimate aim is to persuade us to buy something . . . advertisements must entrap potential customers rapidly and surreptitiously, hitting the brainstem with supernormal stimuli and skirting the reflections of the neocortex. Big, bright and fast replace small, subtle, and mindful.'[10]

This is an interesting reflection about how difficult it is to find out what we really care about in the arts and especially music.

Benjamin Zephaniah makes a similar observation about modern-day popular music when he writes of the restrictions put on the length of music played by the radio stations purely for money-making reasons. He goes on to explain that a good piece of music is created by taking time and care over it. In the present day, if a composer writes anything more than four minutes long, the radio stations won't play it and people won't hear it. What we hear is being controlled by the radio stations. It also means that people are not given the opportunity and time to invest emotionally and thoughtfully in a piece of music. This really contributes to the idea that the arts do not need to be taken seriously. Classic FM plays shorter pieces in general but occasionally a longer piece finds its way through. Some pieces of popular music, however, do shine through the smoke screen of radio station rules because of their intrinsic aesthetic quality, such as *The Closest Thing to Crazy*, sung by Katie Melua and written by Mike Batt. Dissanayake comments on how what we care about deeply as persons, our ultimate concerns, which were traditionally mirrored for us in the arts and religion, are ignored by politicians and business people because these ultimate concerns are un-economic. At this present time, 'having fun' and being superficially entertained is what they spend *our* money on. She writes:

> 'For after the fun and ease and spontaneity pall, when every subsistence need is filled, the ultimate concerns remain. Politicians and business people may tell us that making and experiencing the arts is un-economical and irrelevant for addressing immediate practical problems, but for coming to terms with the human condition we could do far worse than to take the arts seriously.'[11]

References

1 Malloch S (1999) Mothers and infants and communicative musicality. *Musicae Scientiae.* Special Issue 1999–2000. The European Society for Cognitive Sciences, Belgium, p. 48.
2 Zuckerkandl V (1956) *Sound and Symbol.* Bollingen Series XLIV. Princeton University Press, Princeton, NJ, p. 95.
3 Langer S (1942) *Philosophy in a New Key.* Harvard University Press, Cambridge, Mass.
4 De Nora T (2000) *Music in Everyday Life.* Cambridge University Press, Cambridge, p. 53.
5 Dissanayake E (2000) *Art and Intimacy: How the Arts Began.* University of Washington Press, Washington, p. 208.
6 Ibid, p. 209.
7 Ibid, p. 7.
8 Ibid, pp. 209–18.
9 Ibid, p. 216.
10 Ibid, p. 224.
11 Ibid, p. 225.

PART 2

How Do We Understand What We Know?

CHAPTER 6

The philosophy and sociology of the experience of music

Towards a philosophy of music within psychotherapy

At this moment of writing there does not seem to be a philosophy that underpins adequately the experience of music within psychotherapy. This may be because, incredibly as it may appear, until very recently music has been considered as a separate discipline in its own right and not considered as intrinsically part of what it is to be human.

The philosophy of music in the past has dealt mainly with music within itself, its structure and form, and not a lot has been written about the experience of music. What has been written about musical experience has tended to set up a hierarchy in which classical music was considered as 'High Art' and the rest of music was that which was not classical music. There was an interest in folk music, which had a somewhat privileged place in this hierarchy, perhaps because there had been collections of such music by respected musicologists, for example Cecil Sharp or the composer Vaughan Williams. However, what it is to be a human being, experiencing all kinds of music, is now being addressed in the 21st century through many disciplines, notably sociology, psychology, biology and the neurosciences.

In this chapter we will consider some of the writings in the philosophy of music that come nearest to the experience of listening and indeed the playing of music. We will then look at some of the writings on the experience of music from the fields of sociology and psychology. We will consider how cognitive and affective neuroscience contributes to the experience of music in Chapter 7.

Considering the following disciplines will be rather like choosing different threads, which weave into a basic philosophy that will underpin the experience of listening to music within the consulting room. But before looking at these disciplines more closely we will start with what has been written on the universal experience of music.

Music as a universal experience

According to Lucy Green, 'A society without music has never been discovered'.[1] Human beings, it seems, have always made music and of course listened to it. In that sense it is universal. However, the only discrete universals in music that are said to exist are musical sounds, musical conceptualisations and musical behaviour. Musical style is said to be more problematic when it comes to applying the word 'universal' to it. But the simplest worldwide music is said to be songs. These consist of a simple phrase repeated several times with slight variations and only using three or four pitches within the range of a fifth, that is the first five notes of a scale. These forms seem to be universal.[2]

Musical sounds have always existed and human beings have made and listened to them. Fragments of a bone flute have been found at a Mousterian site in Slovenia said to be 4000 years old.[3] But, what is it then that makes music different from the natural sounds we experience, like the lapping of waves on the sea shore or the creaking of branches in the forest?

The answer is to do with being human. It is a human being who takes the tones and also sometimes the sounds that exist and shapes them into forms of feeling, contexts of tones and rhythms. We then perform or listen to these compositions as music.

When we consider only modern Western society, for the moment, the music we experience can range from a simple song or popular jingle through to the increasingly complex ordering of tones and rhythms of modern jazz or a classical symphony. As a complex society we experience, for example, rock music, rap, blues, country and western, reggae, musicals, string quartets, instrumental sonatas, concertos, symphonies, operas and oratorios, etc. Apart from these very different styles of music, human beings also belong to different groupings or cultures within society. Within these groupings there is music for dancing, music at pop concerts, classical concerts, music for ritual and music for solemn occasions as well as everyday music and music in therapy. (We have noted the music for different groupings in our four conversations with people in the public eye, *see* Chapters 1–4.)

These different types of music and cultures of people can be found all over the world as well as within Western society. The music recording industry has greatly contributed to the fact that popular music from all over the world can now be experienced almost anywhere. Less familiar to our ears, however, are the traditional musical compositions of Africa, India, China, Japan, and their different forms of classical music.

The musical composer, then, is situated within an inter-personal context, a social grouping of persons, a human culture. It is therefore not only in Western society that this diversity of styles of music shows itself within different groupings of people; this diversity is worldwide. Ian Cross writes, 'Humans are one single recently emerged species, biologically fairly uniform though culturally diverse'.[4] We must be aware, then, that when we talk about music we are also talking about the songs, musical sounds and compositions of, for example, the Kaluli of Papua New Guinea or the Venda children's songs of Africa. Music in this 21st century is culturally defined in terms of groupings of persons, and although to be a human being is universal, how we express this humanity through music depends to a great extent on our culture.

From the world of neuroscience we learn that our musicality is evident in our earliest babyhood.[5] This musicality within our neuro-biological design meets with our first carer's attentive sounds of engagement and also the sounds from our particular cultural environment. The infant's experiential frame of musical sounds and movements, before and immediately after birth, is the vehicle of engagement with the world and, in return, this engagement begins to shape the newborn infant's brain. If all goes well at birth and we are healthy infants, we seem to be born to respond to sounds and music, and to engage in musical movement and behaviour. Our neuro-biology is primed for music. As Welch writes:

> 'There is a symbiotic relationship between our neurobiological design for musical behaviour and our socio-cultural (and socio-musical) environment. Societal influences are able to shape cortical structure, function and development (of the brain).'[6]

This statement is important as it means that our musicality is inseparable from our early biological make-up and the sound environment we are born into. As we grow as human beings, this early sonic environment contributes to the further processes of our developing minds and our sense of who we are in the world of persons and things.

We will return to this notion of symbiosis, this lack of separation between being human and musicality in Chapter 12. This human musicality is universal in that an infant's predisposition is to be musical. Some modern writers on music and culture, however, explore whether music itself is universal or whether it is culturally determined.[7] But, when we begin to consider the experience of music we shift the ground of the debate. We no longer view music as an isolated study set apart, to be analysed only in its own musical terms nor do we look at music as only defined by its human cultural grouping. Music as an experience becomes linked to the experience of what it is to be a human being throughout the world. Music as a human experience has a universal root in our infancy. But this view also recognises that in sharing what it is to be musical human beings we are also culturally diverse. The experience of music is therefore universal *and* encultured. We will explore more of this philosophical and cultural study of music before we approach the psychological experience of music more directly.

Music and the philosophers

Of the many writers and philosophers on music only those who are nearest to defining the personal *experience* of music will be considered here. This approach is quite different from examining music acoustically within a laboratory or as a phenomenon existing by itself to be studied in terms of its history, key structure and form.

The philosopher Zuckerkandl[8] maintains a universal view on music in that he writes of it as 'motion in the dynamic field of tones' and these tones are framed into music by human beings who join up in some dynamic way with the motion in the dynamic field of tones. This phrase of Zuckerkandl has a great richness in it that will be uncovered as we progress in our search for an underpinning philosophy of musical experience. In particular, he states that this *motion* in music, in this dynamic field of tones, exists in the inner world of the psyche as well as in the outer world of things. He writes:

'There is no doubt that the word "motion" is as native to the inner as to the outer world.'

He continues that this motion is:

'. . . motion which has not been wedded to a body or a psyche (and is) the pureist, most primal form of motion we know. . . . and it is true . . . that at the core of every motion, including the motion of bodies, music lies hidden.'[9]

Here we have a direct philosophical link to music within the dynamic motion in psychotherapy. Motion between the psyches of patient and therapist is central to what we call psychodynamic psychotherapy.

Zuckerkandl goes further when he writes that music provides not only a source of knowledge of the inner world of the psyche but of the world, the cosmos itself.[10] This statement would seem to incorporate all the motion in music, as described through the disciplines of psychology, sociology and neuroscience referred to above.

Susanne Langer focuses on one particular kind of motion in music, that of its dynamic motion as it relates to the inner world of the human psyche. She also takes the view that music is universal in that it is a dynamic *symbol* of the inner life of the emotions. In her view when we engage with music we learn about the forms of feeling which frame the content of our emotional lives. She writes:

'Because the forms of human feeling are much more congruent with musical forms than with forms of language music can *reveal* the nature of feelings with a detail and truth that language cannot approach.'[11]

She describes these forms of feeling as 'patterns of motion and rest, of tension and release, of agreement and disagreement, preparation, fulfilment, excitation, sudden change.'[12] We all have and experience dynamic forms of feeling which are congruent with musical shapes, for example, the motion of the slow build-up of tension at the beginning of Brahms' *First Symphony* which evaporates as it approaches the highest point of tension, but Langer stops short of suggesting how this insight into our inner world of feeling might function therapeutically. However, any psychodynamic psychotherapist recognises these forms or patterns of motion and rest, tension and release, etc. within the consulting room every day. These patterns are present in the way the patient moves and how the therapist might mirror this movement. They are there in the non-verbal communication between them, in the personal narrative of the patient and the therapeutic conversation about this narrative.

But although Zuckerkandl begins to engage with the human experience of music, his view is from the 'outside looking in' on the human mind, an observer's stance on this human experience. Langer's view, however, moves further inside the human experience as she attempts to come to grips with the inner dynamic structures and forms of feeling in the mind as these forms and shapes engage with the experience of music.

Naomi Cumming was a modern thinker whose book *The Sonic Self* also engages with the experiential aspects of music and her writing has informed aspects of this author's thinking on the adult experience of music. More particularly she states that the experience of music is as if the listener or performer is in relation to a person. On the idea of 'getting' a phrase of music, or understanding it emotionally, she writes, 'When such a rapport is established you have not gained a new "concept" but you have gained a new relationship'.[13] The relationship the listener or performer has with the phrase of music is said to be like getting to know someone's special mood or way of being. This notion of dynamic engagement with music and through music to the person of the listener or performer or to 'as if' persons, in Naomi Cumming's thinking, is an experiential strand running through all of these philosophers' writings.

The sociological view

In contrast to the view of these philosophers that music is universal and personal in some dynamic way, some more modern writers on music from a sociological perspective maintain that what exists are 'musics' and not a single phenomenon called music.[7] As such, these 'musics' are seen as totally culturally determined. For example, a Beethoven string quartet on the one hand and the music of the Beatles on the other may be described in terms of the musical forms and structures and be found to be coherent and appropriate to the musical ideas. But when the descriptions of these different pieces of music move beyond this kind of structural analysis, this approach would seem to be reluctant to explore the universal experience of motion in music as it is linked to what it is to be human. This would be to open up the study of the *experience* of motion in music as connected to *individual* motion in the human being. For some sociological studies this would be to move too far towards the individual experience, which is not their remit.

However, they do address the human experience of motion and music in groups. This informs the study of group cultural behaviour that is central to their study of society. Because of this focus on the society or group there is also no consideration of the aesthetic in music as having something universal about it. The idea that there is something about the experience of music that could be considered by all human beings as beautiful or striking would be to confront the post-modern claim that such an experience is *only* culturally defined.

The individual unique aesthetic experience within any culture is considered of great importance in this book. An understanding of the desire for the beautiful or important in music as *a* universal in its psychological depth is glided over in some modern cultural thinking. However, there are exceptions. Tia De Nora, Ellen Dissanayake and Judith Becker are among the exceptions, and each writes on the human being experiencing music and also the desire for the special in music.[14–16] Their thinking will be touched on later. However, the biocultural evolutionary perspective on the experience of music also tries to grasp what is universal among the modern theories of culture.[17]

A biocultural evolutionary perspective on music

Ian Cross writing from a biocultural evolutionary perspective states:

> 'Music is not just universal across cultures; it appears that everyone has the capacity to be musical, though this capacity is likely to be realised to different degrees and in different ways in different cultural and social environments.'[18]

He maintains that in spite of the many cultures that express their identity through music they are all grounded in human behaviours, in other words grounded in what it means to be human. What then are the attributes or characteristics of music which inform us of this human connection?

Cross identifies four universal characteristics of music which connect it with human evolution. He writes that music has not only involved sound but action.

> 'Any attempt to find human attributes of music must acknowledge the embodied nature of music, the indivisibility of movement and sound in characterizing music across histories and societies.'[19]

We have only to watch or take part in a modern pop concert to be aware of the physical movement that is inseparable from the music performed to recognise this characteristic in action.

The second connection between music and persons is that a piece of music can bear multiple meanings at the same time. He refers to Feld's description of a piece of music as functioning as a communication with the dead for the Kaluli of Papua New Guinea and 'binding birds, souls, places and people at a time of transformation'.[20] A modern example of how a piece of music can bear multiple meanings at the same time is how people 'understand' the experience of a piece of classical music quite differently. The piece of music is capable of carrying several feelings at once, such as joy and grief together.

The third characteristic which informs us of the human connection with music is that it is grounded in social interaction and personalised meaning. Cross gives an example of music in social interaction within a culture by quoting Blacking's work referring to music used in restructuring social relations in the domba initiation of the Venda tribe. Blacking himself writes of this restructuring of social relations through music as follows:

> 'Beer songs whose words allow wife-givers and wife-takers systematically to exchange formal, and often ribald, complaints about each other's perform- ance of the duties associated with their relationship.'[21]

Any public ceremony today does seem to demand that music contains and helps to structure social interaction. The opening ceremony of the Olympic Games comes to mind here. It is difficult to think of such an occasion without music being available to shape the social interaction and give focus to the general meaning, the national pride and celebration of achievement at such an event. Also, when the winning athlete stands on the podium and the national flag is raised, the personalised meaning of their National Anthem, the sense of pride, the sense of belonging etc. is shown in the athlete's face.

The fourth attribute of music, according to Cross, is that it has no particular survival value. He writes that music can neither provide food nor kill enemies. But he introduces the idea of 'muscular bonding'.[22] This occurs within a group of people where communal feeling experience is elicited by moving together rhythmically to music. Cross goes on to say that this rhythmic synchronicity promotes group identity and enhanced co-operative survival strategies in, for example, a hunting expedition or in battle between warring groups. The Maori rugby *Haka* chant before a game would certainly be said to promote group identity.

Cross then traces back the rhythmic synchronicity that promotes group identity to Colwyn Trevarthen's work on the musicality of infant–mother interaction and its 'time-sharing' capacities.[23] These capacities are there to promote bonding and attunement between infant and mother. According to Trevarthen and Malloch the musical communication between infant and mother at this level of bodily expression 'has a fundamental role in the genesis of human well-being and the nurturance of "belonging" in a community'.[5] This is then an evolutionary *reason*, according to Cross, for music to exist in human culture. He writes further that:

> 'If evolution has shaped the human mind, it has most likely selected at the level of infant predispositions, and culture can be thought of as shaping into specific and distinct forms the expression of these predispositions.'[24]

To sum up, Cross highlights the importance of music and movement synchro- nicity between groups, and the various meanings music can hold for groups of persons, along with music's importance in social interaction which he traces back to Trevarthen's work with infant–mother communicative musicality. He does not however focus particularly on the *dynamic* musical motion between infant and mother nor does he address the more intimate interpersonal *dynamics* in musical contexts. In this sense, it is still an arm's length approach.

It is the writing of Tia De Nora, *Music in Everyday Life*, that takes a step nearer to exploring this dynamic motion between persons through music, which is the focus of music within psychotherapy.[25] She describes her approach to this sociological enquiry as ethnographic. This means that she explores the dynamic of *how* the individual experiences and makes sense of music in social interactions within groups of persons.

An ethnographical approach

Tia De Nora considers and examines different styles of music listened to by people in their everyday lives.[26] She provides accounts of music's structuring power in everyday experiences, such as music used in an aerobics class, a karaoke evening and active music therapy sessions with percussion. She focuses on what music is as a resource and what it does in these situations. In particular she identifies ways in which we use music in the care of self. She suggests that we use music as a resource which we turn to for exploration of the 'self' and regulation of this 'self'. We are said to manage who we are through music so that we function in a good enough way in the world and have a sense of agency. By this sense of agency she may mean a cognitive choice about what we want to hear in order to feel relaxed or get into the party spirit. She gives examples of interviewees choosing music to prepare for going out for the evening or choosing music to set the mood for a cocktail party or barbecue.

In another research study De Nora describes the day-to-day lives of American and British women and how they use music 'to regulate, enhance and change qualities and levels of emotion'.[27] This research is indeed very valuable as it shows how some of us use music to regulate our moods if there is either not too much disturbance to our sense of self and sense of self-in-relationship, or if perhaps there is too much disturbance of our sense of self-in-relationship and we use music to dissociate from who we are and what we are really feeling about our 'selves'.

But this day-to-day care of self and *self-regulation* is not what is being addressed in listening to music within psychotherapy. With the patient in the consulting room the sense of self-in-relationship of the patient has been owned by them as a troubled self-in-relationship. The therapist understands that they are working with a person who is not yet in a comfortable place psychologically as a self-in-relationship. They may be fragile, disorganised and avoidant in relationship with other persons.

This psychological terrain is very different from that described in De Nora's book. De Nora notes this qualitative difference herself when she describes mùsic's powers as being capable of extending beyond its capacity for change for the listener on a short-term basis. She sees clearly that music has the capacity to be more than a quick fix and resource for mood change. She writes:

'Its temporal dimension, the fact that it is a non-verbal, non-depictive medium, and that it is a physical presence whose vibrations can be felt, all enhance its ability to work at non-cognitive or subconscious levels.'[28]

This work at non-cognitive or subconscious levels would indeed describe music within psychotherapy. Although she does not explore this discipline further she articulates the terrain when she describes music as a way of happening. She writes:

> 'Music is not "about" anything but is rather a material that happens over time and in particular ways. Music is a medium, *par excellence*, of showing us how happening may occur.'[29]

Of the several ways music can be described as happening (listened to or created), she notes that music can be 'One against many, all together, fugal, homophonic, softly, loudly, gentle or abrupt, legato, staccato, relaxed, or tense'.[20] These ways of happening are reminiscent of Susanne Langer's forms of feeling in the world of the philosophy of music mentioned above. These forms of feeling, which are said to be the structures of our inner mental life include relaxed, abrupt, gentle. staccato, legato, sudden etc.[30] They also correspond to Stern's vitality affects, the psychological ways of engagement which he has identified in early infant/mother communication.[31] We will return to these ways of being and forms and happening in music in our inner mental world later in the case study with Liz (*see* Chapter 10).

However, what is most relevant to listening to music within psychotherapy is how De Nora describes how we use music in the 'care of self' within her cognitive frame of reference. There would seem to be an overlap here between the ethnographic interview and the beginnings of a psychotherapeutic process.

She writes in *Music in Everyday Life* that we first use music as a resource to turn to for exploration of the 'self' and its regulation, that is how we *manage* who we are so that we function in a 'good enough' way in the world and have a sense of agency. We next use music to discover *who* we are subjectively in mind and body that is, our experience as human selves. De Nora then presents a third way in which we use music which is the stories we tell ourselves and others which provides us with a narrative of our being and doing in the world.[32]

This ethnographic approach is similar to the interviews at the beginning of this book, in which we read of the interviewees' accounts of what music meant for each of them. As has been said, these interviews were not psychotherapeutic sessions even though there were nuances of such sessions. The interviewees were listened to carefully and empathised with. My own opinions, thoughts and feelings were kept mostly to myself. This in itself would have had a mild therapeutic effect in that each interviewee was given space to tell his or her own story and hear, through my reflection and confirmation of their own words, their own sense of self-in-relationship and agency.

These descriptions of how we use music and the connections to who we are as individuals goes some way to mapping out what is going on in music used as a medium in psychotherapy. But De Nora is well aware of the limitations of using music only within a cognitive framework, which denies the impact of the subconscious mind. She writes:

'Such a conception (the cognivist conception of agency) stops short of the more profound levels on which music also operates, the levels on which we do not turn to music as a resource but are rather caught up in it, find ourselves in the middle of it. Are awakened by it.'[28]

By saying that we are awakened by music, De Nora could be describing what happens for the patients listening to music within psychotherapy sessions, as will be described later in this book. In such a session music is used as a medium in which both patient and therapist are caught up and find themselves in relation within it. What is markedly different is that what is being explored by De Nora is 'care of self' and self-regulation and what is being focused on in listening to music within the psychotherapy sessions is 'care of self-in-relationship'. Here the patient chooses the music and discovers aspects of who they are in relationship. The centre of the enquiry is not the elusive 'self' that De Nora attempts to describe but an equally elusive self-in-relationship. Apart from this point, the description of the 'care of self' from her cognitive perspective of personal encounters with listening to music would fit quite easily into the psychodynamic frame of what happens in the consulting room with the patient. But there is more going on in this psychotherapeutic encounter with music than is addressed here and we will now consider psychological aspects of music and psychology to widen our understanding.

References

1 Green L (2003) Music education, cultural capital and social group identity. In: M Clayton, T Herbert and R Middleton (eds) *Cultural Study of Music*. Routledge, New York and London, p. 263.
2 Nettl B (2000) An ethnomusicologist contemplates universals in musical sound and musical culture. In: N Wallin, B Merker and S Brown (eds) *The Origins of Music*. MIT Press, Cambridge, Mass., p. 469.
3 Kunej D and Turk I (2000) New perspectives on the beginnings of music: archeological and musicological analysis of a middle pateolithic bone 'flute'. In: N Wallin, B Merker and S Brown (eds) *The Origins of Music*. MIT Press, Cambridge, Mass., p. 235.
4 Cross I (2003) Music and biocultural evolution. In: M Clayton, T Herbert and R Middleton (eds) *The Cultural Study of Music*. Routledge, New York and London, p. 21.
5 Trevarthen C and Malloch S (2002) The musical lives of babies and families. *Journal of Zero to Three: National Center for Infants Toddlers and Families*. 23(1): 11.
6 Welch G (2001) *The Misunderstanding of Music*. Institute of Education, University of London, p. 7.
7 Clayton M, Herbert T and Middleton R (eds) (2003) *The Cultural Study of Music*. Routledge, New York and London.
8 Zuckerkandl V (1956) *Sound and Symbol*. Bollingen Series XLIV. Princeton University Press, Princeton, NJ, p.143.
9 Ibid, pp. 143–5.

10 Ibid, p. 147.

11 Langer S (1942) *Philosophy in a New Key.* Harvard University Press, Cambridge, Mass., p. 235. (Reprinted 1996).

12 Ibid, p. 228.

13 Cumming N (2000) *The Sonic Self.* Indiana University Press, Bloomington, Indianapolis, p. 222.

14 De Nora T (2000) *Music in Everyday Life.* Cambridge University Press, Cambridge.

15 Dissanayake E (2000) *Art and Intimacy.* University of Washington Press, Washington.

16 Becker J (2004) *Deep Listeners.* Indiana University Press, Bloomington, Indianapolis.

17 Cross I (2003) Music and biocultural evolution. In: M Clayton, T Herbert and R Middleton (eds) *The Cultural Study of Music.* Routledge, New York and London.

18 Cross I (2003) Music, cognition, culture and evolution. In: I Peretz and R Zatorre (eds) *The Cognitive Neuroscience of Music.* Oxford University Press, Oxford, p. 47.

19 Cross I (2003) *The Cultural Study of Music.* Routledge, New York and London, p. 23.

20 Feld S (1990) Sound and sentiment. Birds weeping poetics and song in Kaluli experience. University of Pennsylvania Press. Quoted in: M Clayton, T Herbert and R Middleton (eds) (2003) *The Cultural Study of Music.* Routledge, New York and London, p. 23.

21 Blacking J (1973) *Music, Culture and Experience.* University of Chicago Press, Chicago, p. 40.

22 Mcneill WH (1995) Keeping together in time. Harvard University Press, London. Quoted in: I Peretz and R Zatorre (eds) (2003) The *Cognitive Neuroscience of Music.* Oxford University Press, Oxford, p. 5.

23 Trevarthen C (1999) Musicality and the intrinsic motive pulse: evidence from human psycho-biology and infant communication. *Musicae Scientiae.* Special Issue 1999–2000. The European Society for Cognitive Sciences, Belgium, p. 155.

24 Cross I (2003) Music and biocultural evolution. In: M Clayton, T Herbert and R Middleton (eds) *The Cultural Study of Music.* Routledge, New York and London, p. 25.

25 De Nora T (2000) *Music in Everyday Life.* Cambridge University Press, Cambridge, pp. 38–40.

26 Ibid, p. 46.

27 De Nora T (2001) Aesthetic agency and musical practice: new directions in the sociology of music and emotion. In: P Juslin and J Sloboda (eds) *Music and Emotion.* Oxford University Press, Oxford, p. 169.

28 De Nora T (2000) *Music in Everyday Life.* Cambridge University Press, Cambridge, p. 159.

29 Ibid, p. 158.

30 Langer S (1942) *Philosophy in a New Key.* Harvard University Press, Cambridge, Mass., p. 228. Reprinted 1996.

31 Stern D (1985) *The Interpersonal World of the Infant.* Basic Books, USA, pp. 53–61.

32 De Nora T (2000) *Music in Everyday Life.* Cambridge University Press, Cambridge, Mass., pp. 158–60.

CHAPTER 7

The psychology of the experience of music

Juslin and Sloboda's writing in *Music and Emotion* has much that is relevant to thinking about music in psychotherapy. It focuses on different types of studies of music and emotion within society, moving nearer still to exploring listening to music within psychotherapy. What are not addressed of course are the non-verbal in-depth dimensions of psychotherapeutic understanding nor the idea of interpersonal emotional psychodynamic engagement through listening to music together within therapy. They do, however, highlight that emotion is deeply connected with music and that the study of these connections has been sidestepped in the past. They write:

> 'Appreciation of music is often taken to mean having an intellectual under-standing of the history and form of a musical composition rather than an articulated emotional response.'[1]

Sloboda and O'Neill observe, however, that the psychological approach to the study of music and emotion has also in the past tended to ignore the social context of musical behaviour, which they state is 'enmeshed in a social and cultural world.'[2] This is an interesting point for reflection in the context of music in psychotherapy and music throughout the Health Service. It could be said to be a caution against any psychotherapeutic technique that concentrates on an interpretation of the inner musical experience of the patient to the exclusion of the social context of their engagement with music. This social context could be the patient with their friends and family and how music is experienced in these dynamic contexts, and also the inter-subjective dynamic relationship with the therapist and what the chosen music means for the patient here. It could also mean the wider social contexts of concerts or musical happenings where an audience is present. They write:

> 'The impact of music and emotion is not direct but interdependent on the situations in which it is heard. Any meaningful account of music's role in the emotional response of individuals must involve the recognition of these complex interdependent social factors.'[3]

This statement also has important implications for music heard in a general healthcare situation and must be considered in waiting areas in hospitals, GP surgeries, etc. Are anxious listeners irritated by the music played perhaps? Might it not increase their heart rate and blood pressure in unhelpful ways? Perhaps the visual mode only should be available so that they could ignore the visual if they wanted to rather than having to listen to intrusive music, from which they cannot easily escape because of appointments made. There is much exploration of the arts in health at present and such visual ideas could well be adopted in GP surgeries that would not involve the intrusive aspects of imposed music. If, more particularly, the impact of music and emotion is interdependent on the situation in which it is heard, music within psychotherapy has other psychological features that must be considered. We will now turn to significant psychological enquiries that will inform listening to music within psychotherapy.

Everyday uses of music

In the book *Music and Emotion*, in the research chapter on 'The everyday uses of music', music is described as ubiquitous in contemporary life and most of what we encounter as listeners is said by definition to be mundane. The contexts in which we encounter such music include 'waking up, washing and dressing, eating, cleaning, shopping, travelling.'[3] In this chapter the authors attend carefully to the contexts in which the music is listened to and exclude the special times of emotional significance in which we encounter music. Although these special times may be very significant in defining the relationship between music and emotion Sloboda and O'Neill hold the view that 'it is the everyday and normal which frames and helps to define the special.'[3]

The method used by Sloboda and O'Neill was the experience sampling method (ESM) in which the participants carried electric pagers with them at all times during waking hours. The participants were paged once every two hours between 0800 and 2200 hours. They were asked to stop what they were doing when appropriate and write responses in a booklet regarding the most recent experience of listening to music since they were last paged. This could be on the radio or in a shop, etc. This piece of research is different from most in the field of psychology and music in that those persons who were the human experiencing subjects did not have to listen to music chosen by the researcher. However, they did not have complete control over the particular music listened to either.

This notion of the mundane in music defining the framework of the special, however, is explored further in this book. The outline framing of the experiences of mundane music will be used to shape a pathway or route from the exterior observable world of social psychology to the hidden interior world of non-verbal musical encounter within psychotherapy. This outline framing will be identified through key features, which Sloboda and O'Neill have used in their research, which describe a more human and personal encounter with music that is different from research that takes place in a laboratory setting. These key features, which will be said to shape this pathway are:

- Autonomy and individuality.
- Personal and social identity.
- Music as self-therapy.

Examples of extremely intense and sometimes transcendental experiences which people characterise as life changing are included in *Music and Emotion* in Gabrielssohn's chapter, 'Emotions in strong experiences with music'.[4] We will address these intense experiences later alongside the work of others including De Nora, Becker and Dissanayake.[5-7] For the moment, we will briefly describe the study on 'everyday experiences of music' using categories of the research as signposts to construct a framework which will embrace not only mundane musical experiences but also the more special musical experiences.

Autonomy and individuality – the first signpost

What is most interesting for 'music within psychotherapy' is that Sloboda and O'Neill discovered that in terms of autonomy and individuality, the greater the choice of music the greater the change in the participant's mood.[8] They found that music in low choice situations occurred mainly with others, in shops, in gyms and in engaging in an activity because one really wants to do it. It would seem that really wanting to engage in a particular activity overcame the lack of personal musical choice. High choice situations were most likely to occur when the person was alone, travelling or working at home or undertaking activities for duty. They suggest that choosing music to accompany duties was a way of bringing some autonomy back to the individual.

This finding on personal choice of music being linked to change in the participant's mood in the above situations has implications for listening to music within psychotherapy. The patient's choice of music would seem to be important even for mundane music, let alone music which is *really important* for them. There are of course exceptions. In Guided Imagery and Music (GIM) the therapist, after much intensive training, chooses the music but the patient group with which such music therapists usually engage is very different from that usually encountered within word-based psychotherapy.

Patients in such groups may be suffering from cerebral palsy or other severe neurological or psychological impairment and they may not be in an appropriate mental or neurological place to make a choice of which music to listen to. This will be discussed more fully later. It will, however, be suggested here that if the patient is able to choose the music, this should be the preferred method within psychotherapy as it is radically non-intrusive and preserves the patient's autonomy in circumstances where this autonomy feels under threat. One example from psychotherapeutic practice to be discussed more fully later is that of Liz. After several years of conventional psychotherapy she was attending a pain clinic for treatment of fibromyalgia, when she realised that very painful mental states were being tapped into which she could not contain. Talking through this with her consultant she decided to come back into therapy and chose to listen to music as a method of working.

This moved her on quite quickly as will be seen from her case study in Chapter 10.

Personal and social identity – the second signpost

The second set of features which moves closer to the terrain of psychotherapy is personal and social identity. Here the authors found that music is a kind of mirror through which the listener interprets who they are. They write:

> 'Music provides numerous ways in which musical materials and practices can be used as a means of self-interpretation, self presentation, and for the expression of emotional states, associated with the self.'[9]

This sentence could describe, in general terms, a good reason for the practice of using listening to music within psychotherapy.

However, within their particular discipline, Sloboda and O'Neill write here of the importance of the period of adolescence in monitoring the thread of the emotional self through music. They write that 81% of young people say that music is an important part of their lives and influences how they think about important issues according to Leming.[10] This is said to be in direct contrast to watching TV, which adolescents do not believe has had a major influence in their lives.[11] Larson *et al.* are quoted as finding that music listening was associated with greater personal involvement than TV watching, which was associated with feeling less happy, less alert, more passive and more bored than at other times.[12]

A further interesting piece of research is quoted by North *et al.* who found that there were marked gender differences in adolescents' reasons for listening to music.[13] It seems that girls use music mainly for mood regulation, an inner mental activity, whilst boys use music as a means of creating an external impression with their peers. What is particularly interesting here is that even although the reason boys listened to music was to impress others, they tended to listen to it privately. 'Thus the external impression the boys sought to accomplish did not necessarily involve direct social contact at the time they were actively listening to music.' This is interpreted as the boys being actively involved in the construction of their identity rather than changing their mood. They did this through stereotypes and gender role models associated with the music they listened to. In other words, they were more influenced by the 'macho and sexy image of male pop/rock musicians playing mainly guitars and drums' rather than the music itself.[13]

Using music within psychotherapy teaches us that a patient's musical experiences described at the time of adolescence are very significant as they may offer much information and understanding about who the patient wanted to be and might still want to be in terms of self-identity. One patient, Thomas, recalled that playing rock music during his adolescence was when he discovered, for the first time, a strong sense of self-identity and self-confidence in relationships. This was an important recollection to return to and re-experience in the consulting room.

The research by Sloboda and O'Neill is significant but it is suggested here that this thread of a sense of self and sense of self-in-relation would first arise in infancy through what Trevarthen and Malloch have called 'communicative musicality'.[14]

When musical behaviour is observed in adolescence it will have its roots in these patterns of communicative musicality through early attachment with an important carer or carers, usually the mother. How psychodynamic and psycho-analytic psychotherapists begin to understand the inner world of the person in the consulting room is by considering the development in relationship of the growing infant and child with their first carers. The patient's musical prefer-ences and how they used music in adolescence may be noted by the psy-chotherapist, as will the narrative of their relationship to music as they mature. Is the patient using music to hide in and not face interpersonal relationships in the world? Or is he or she able to use music to enjoy life and use it as an acceptable medium to engage interpersonally with others, for example at a rock concert or folk group.

In the consulting room the transference attachment, that is the intense feeling or feelings experienced by the patient towards the therapist, may reach back to an earlier troubled attachment pattern with the mother or first carer, which may be revisited through music. Music in this context might be a place to escape to for the client to avoid embarrassing loving feelings they now have for the therapist. We have the example of James, a patient of a colleague, who brought in a tape of a love song at the end of the joint psychotherapeutic work. This work will be described more fully in Chapter 14.

In another situation this avoidance of powerful feeling(s) towards the person or the therapist might indicate a pattern of dissociation into music. Here, the patient might experience a trance-like state, which again would be in avoidance of strong feelings that they are unable to manage with words. These strong feelings may also originate from times of early inter-personal trauma in the patient's life and there may be indications that the patient is not in touch with their body either.

Ways in which the patient uses music in the consulting room will be seen in the case study material discussed in later chapters. For example, Liz listened with me to a piece of music of her own choice. It was a passage from a Dvorak symphony. She next recalled an experience when she was about six years old. This was, according to her, the first time she remembered feeling close to her mother. There was then a memory of sitting next to her mother on a bus and experiencing the warm texture of her coat and the feeling of being tenderly cared for. These would be examples of displacement of warm feelings into music, feelings that were perhaps too intense and experienced too early to be verba-lised. These intense feelings might also have had a shadow side which again could not be expressed in words but which could have been dissociated from the warm feelings experienced in the music. This will be discussed more fully in Chapter 12.

There was also Peter, an earlier patient, who was suddenly aware of his creative self-in-relationship whilst playing a recording of his own composed music in the consulting room with me. He had lost sight of this young energetic Peter and had little sense of who he really was before this session. Because of his early infant experience of the traumatic loss of his mother and other indications of him not being bodily present in the world, music could have been used in his life to cover, as it were, the break or traumatic loss of his mother. It provided him with a sense of going-on-being when this traumatic feeling of complete loss arose in his mind. We will now turn to Sloboda and O'Neill's third feature of music as self-therapy.

Music as self-therapy – the third signpost

Sloboda and O'Neill consider the idea of everyday music as self-therapy. They show evidence that music is used deliberately to achieve psychological outcomes which are then seen to bring about emotional change. But as they themselves note, therapy as understood and practised by therapists is not just about the manipulation of emotions; it is about helping an individual to manage life's difficulties and find a more appropriate way of being in the world and relating to other people. They do acknowledge that there is nothing in the literature on everyday music uses that brings about the kinds of changes that help solve personal problems, or evidence that music helps to find the inner resources to assist in making difficult decisions. But they go on to say that there is strong anecdotal evidence by users of music that such effects do exist, but the mechanisms by which these effects are mediated are poorly theorised. They suggest however that 'everyday' psychological disorders such as 'depression' may be helped by well-chosen pieces of music. They write:

> 'Well chosen pieces of music might be able to help individuals break out of such cycles by the specific combination of intrinsic and extrinsic cues that they provide.'[15]

Apart from seriously interfering with the personal autonomy of someone suffering from an 'everyday' psychological disorder of depression as it is described, this raises the question of who chooses the music and in what context. This method of working described by Sloboda and O'Neill would not be the one chosen in music in psychotherapy with such patients. It would be felt to be important that the personal autonomy was preserved and that they decide whether to listen to music or not and also what kind of music. The patient's choice of music would seem to be essential.

It will now be becoming clear that music within psychotherapy is a quite different form of therapy from the research discussed above into music as self-therapy. Although the individual persons in the research are interviewed by a respectful researcher, the music is the primary focus, not the *relationship* between the person of the researcher and the person of the interviewee. Music takes centre stage in Sloboda and O'Neill's method of enquiry, as it were, and persons-in-relationship are in the background. They do, however, acknowledge that interpersonal relationships *are* there in any musical scenario. They write:

'It is a significant feature of the emotional feelings and displays that individuals experience in relation to the everyday musical scenarios that we have outlined that although they may occur in solitude, their point of reference is the relationship between the music user and others. Although viewed as essentially "private", experiences involving a great deal of autonomy or agency, emotional feelings and displays are deeply embedded in a social context, which exerts a powerful influence (albeit often implicitly) on our music listening.'[16]

Within the medium of music in psychotherapy there is an involvement of the self-in-relationship of the patient and the self-in-relationship of the therapist. Their therapeutic relationship is worked through in the sometime context of shared listening to music chosen by the patient. The aim of this involvement is the repair and restoration of aspects of the self-in-relationship for the patient, which are not functioning well. This special kind of encounter between patient and therapist could be said to be described in its complexity by Becker as the 'habitus of listening to music'. Becker could be describing the complexity of just this special kind of encounter between patient and psychotherapist when she writes:

'Emotional responses to music do not occur spontaneously nor naturally, but rather take place within complex systems of thoughts and behaviour concerning what music means, what it is for, how it is to be perceived and what might be appropriate kinds of expressive responses.'[17]

But as has been already noted above, Sloboda and O'Neill's reason for exploring music as mundane is to throw into relief the important facets of music as special. We will now consider briefly music as special from a psychological perspective, which still, however, focuses on music and not on the person-in-relationship.

Music as special

In *Music and Emotion* Gabrielssohn explores emotion in 'strong experiences of music'. Given that this is not therapeutic research, where there are two people engaged in psychotherapeutic endeavour through the medium of music, this research has interesting aspects. It was based on 400 reports obtained from 300 persons, many providing two or more results. Sixty percent of participants were aged between 20 and 40 and about 30% were aged between 40 and 60. Musical preferences were spread over the generations. The subjects were asked to describe 'the strongest, most intense experience of music you have ever had' and to describe these experiences and reactions in as much detail as they could.[18] The reports were obtained by means of interview and mostly as written reports.

 Even though the above research is concerned with emotional responses to strong experiences of music, which is chosen and listened to by the individual person, it seems very distant and different from the practice of music within psychotherapy. Gabrielssohn himself notes that:

'The focus here has been on emotional aspects of SEM (strong experiences of music) supplemented by some brief outlooks to other aspects and influencing factors.'[19]

He goes on to write that this research project:

'Represents but a limited part of the available material on SEM. Cutting out a part of a whole invariably leads to gaps and imperfections, and the loss of relevant connections of a broader context.'[20]

As such it must be considered a partial exploration of strong experiences of music. One important aspect is that it is self-focused and does not take into account the self-in-relationship.

This being said, there are interesting observations that should be noted in any exploration of music within psychotherapy. For example Gabrielssohn explores emotions in SEM (strong experiences of music) as positive, negative and mixtures of positive and negative that are conflicting.[21]

This latter category was very evident in much of the music brought in by patients within the consulting room with me. As will be seen later in Chapter 10, in Liz's choice of music, the joy and sadness together in her memory of the passage from the Dvorak symphony is an example of this conflicting experience. Then there was Thomas who in his inner pain displayed a traumatic splitting of two inner states in his being-in-relationship. These states were literally 'played out' in the consulting room through the medium of shared listening to music. One piece of music made him feel that he should 'pull his socks up' and 'get over it' and the other piece of music called powerfully to him to 'be still'. Attempts to integrate these conflicting ways of being in the one person-in-relationship was an important strand of the psychotherapeutic work for both of these patients.

Another interesting observation by Gabrielssohn is that the experiences of SEM came from very different musical genres. 'Art' music was the choice of half of the people involved in the research, the other half choosing between pop or rock, jazz, folk music and popular ballads. SEM could occur with any music according to Gabrielssohn. However, it must be said that it would be difficult to imagine strong positive emotions in response to a telephone jingle! It would be easier to recall a strong negative response here. But it is possible that there could be an association with a loving relationship for the listener. This would of course be discovered within psychotherapy! At the end of this research it is stated that:

'In consideration of the ever present interactions between musical, personal and situational factors it may be appropriate to speak of strong experiences *of and with* music or strong experiences *in connection with* music.'[19]

This quotation comes very near to recommending that the person-in-relationship be put in the centre of future research. What would be explored is how it is that they have a strong emotional experience in connection with music. Music in psychotherapy would seem to be the terrain for such an exploration.

Another aspect of music as special is its relationship to time within the context of psychotherapy. We will end this chapter by touching on this important time experience when listening to music within psychotherapy.

The experience of time within music in psychotherapy

The situation of psychotherapy involves long-term or shorter-term work. Within long-term work there are at least two kinds of time experiences which must be considered. The first involves the therapist and patient in present time and the second is to do with past time for the patient. The first one is straightforward in that patient and therapist listen to the music together in real time and share the experience, and comment on it as appropriate. The music has been chosen by the patient. It is music that is understood as music that the patient needs to listen to with a companion. The therapist in this instance is the companion and notes any movement and bodily expression in the patient as well as feeling the music.

In the second experience of time, the therapist should consider the context of the patient's first experience of the chosen music. This would usually be earlier in life. This is then explored if appropriate and the feeling, content and expression noted and empathised with. There are therefore at least two parallel times to be considered. The first personal time is the intersubjective encounter with the therapist in the present, and the second time is remembered time for the patient which is brought into the present through the shared medium of music. These two overlapping times are not addressed in depth in the field of social psychology. They are, however, acknowledged as existing but they are not engaged with in terms of working through their therapeutic significance. This is an appropriate exclusion as this thinking is particular to psychotherapy. However, from the perspective of social psychology, Sloboda and O'Neill enquired of 70 individuals what their early memories of music were:

> 'Seventy individuals were asked to recall any incidents from the first ten years of life that were in any way connected with music. This period was chosen because a major aim of the study was to find connections between early music and later attitudes to music.'[22]

They were asked what meaning and significance the event had for them and each incident was assigned a value on two dimensions. What Sloboda and O'Neill describe as an 'internal dimension' was concerned with *musical content* and an 'external dimension' was to do with context.

On a first reading of this research it might seem that this was the territory of listening to music within psychotherapy, but on closer examination the 'internal dimension' that was investigated was to do with the *musical* content. In listening to music within psychotherapy, the 'internal dimension' is to do with the dynamic motion of *persons* or selves-in-relationship, engaging with each other through the medium of music. It is the dynamic field of persons as it overlaps with the dynamic field of listening to music together. De Nora comes nearer this recognition of the inner experience of *persons* and *music* when she writes:

> 'The study of human-music interaction thus reveals the subject, memory and, with it, self identity, as being constituted on a fundamental socio-cultural plane. . . . Music may thus be seen to serve as a container for the temporal structure of past circumstances. Moreover, to the extent that, first time through, a past event was constructed and came to be meaningful with reference to music, musical structures may provide a grid or grammar for the temporal structures of emotional and embodied patterns as they were originally experienced.'[23]

Here we have an approach that recognises how the experience of being a self and the experience of listening to music overlap. However, although De Nora is very near describing the experience of listening to music within psychotherapy, a further state of being-in-relationship is suggested as occurring within listening to music within the psychotherapeutic framework. Listening to music within psychotherapy occupies a terrain in which the self-in-relationship of the therapist and the self-in-relationship of the patient encounter each other through the medium of the shared flowing container of heard music. Layers of time, such as present time in the consulting room and remembered time, overlap in the shared listening to passages of music chosen by the patient and we will return to these complex ways of being-in-relationship in later chapters.

For the moment, the terrain of social psychology is mainly in the present or, as is described by Sloboda and O'Neill, as being in 'real time', and this discipline does not generally give prominence to what might be called 'remembered time' and its significant influence on the mind. Zuckerkandl, however, noted that music is an auditory image of time. He writes:

> 'Tones are time become audible matter; to form in tones is to form in the stuff of time: an image composed of tones is always at the same time a time image – not an image *in* time but an image made of time. . . . Time and tone completely fill each other – there is literally no room for emptiness.'[24]

When patient and therapist listen to passages of music chosen by the patient there is no space for emptiness, not even the emptiness of remembered loss for the patient. The loss may be remembered when the music ends but the emptiness will be said to be filled with the presence of the therapist and the trace in the patient's brain of early patterns of the mother/carer–infant nurturing relationship, that is, this first musical patterning, this 'communicative musicality'. This will be discussed more fully later in this book in relation to the therapeutic casework with Liz.

Tia De Nora has already been noted for her ethnographic approach to examining the whole experience of music and persons in her exploration of different styles of music listened to by people in their everyday lives. She has more to write about music that is significantly different from everyday music and in the next chapter we will explore further this special kind of musical experience.

References

1   Juslin P and Sloboda J (eds) (2001) *Music and Emotion*. Oxford University Press, Oxford, p. 5.
2   Sloboda J and O'Neill S (2001) Emotions in everyday listening to music. In: P Juslin and J Sloboda (eds) *Music and Emotion*. Oxford University Press, Oxford, p. 428.
3   Ibid, p. 415.
4   Gabrielssohn A (2001) Emotions in strong experiences with music. In: P Juslin and J Sloboda (eds) *Music and Emotion*. Oxford University Press, Oxford, p. 431.
5   De Nora T (2000) *Music in Everyday Life*. Cambridge University Press, Cambridge.
6   Becker J (2004) *Deep Listeners*. Indiana University Press, Bloomington, Indianapolis.
7   Dissanayake E (2000) *Art and Intimacy*, University of Washington Press, Seattle and London.
8   Sloboda J and O'Neill S (2001) Emotions in everyday listening to music. In: P Juslin and J Sloboda (eds) *Music and Emotion*. Oxford University Press, Oxford, p. 421.
9   Ibid, p. 423.
10 Leming J (1987) Rock music and the socialisation of moral values in early adolescence. *Youth and Society*. **18:** 363–83. Quoted in: P Juslin and J Sloboda (eds) *Music and Emotion*. Oxford University Press, Oxford. p. 424.
11 McCormack J (1984) Formative life experiences and the channelling of adolescent goals. Unpublished doctoral dissertation. University of Chicago, Chicago. Quoted in: P Juslin and J Sloboda (eds) *Music and Emotion*. Oxford University Press, Oxford, p. 424.
12 Larson R *et al.* (1989) Changing channels: early adolescent media choices and shifting investments in family and friends. *Journal of Youth and Adolescence.* **18**: 583–600.
13 North A *et al.* (2000) The importance of music to adolescents. *British Journal of Educational Psychology*. **70:** 255–72.
14 Trevarthen C and Malloch S (2002) The musical lives of babies and families. *Journal of Zero to Three: National Center for Infants, Toddlers and Families*. **23**(1): 11.
15 Sloboda J and O'Neill S (2001) Emotions in everyday listening to music. In: P Juslin and J Sloboda (eds) *Music and Emotion*. Oxford University Press, Oxford. p. 426.
16 Ibid, p. 427.
17 Becker J (2001) Anthropological perspectives on music and emotion. In: P Juslin and J Sloboda (eds) *Music and Emotion*. Oxford University Press, Oxford, p. 137.
18 Gabrielssohn A (2001) Emotions in strong experiences with music. In: P Juslin and J Sloboda (eds) *Music and Emotion*. Oxford University Press, Oxford, p. 434.
19 Ibid, p. 445.
20 Ibid, p. 446.
21 Ibid, p. 435.
22 Sloboda J and O'Neill (2001) Emotions in everyday listening to music. In: P Juslin and J Sloboda (eds) *Music and Emotion*. Oxford University Press, Oxford, p. 425.
23 De Nora T (2000) *Music in Everyday Life*. Cambridge University Press, Cambridge, pp. 67–8.

24 Zuckerkandl V (1956) *Sound and Symbol.* Bollingen Series XL1V. Princeton University Press, Princeton NJ, p. 258. (Reprinted 1973).

CHAPTER 8

The 'habitus' of the experience of music and music therapy

The 'habitus' of music

Moving nearer still to exploring listening to music within psychotherapy, we must be more clear about the context of the meeting between patient and psychotherapist. We are not studying the experience of one person only; there are two people involved. However, according to Becker musical scholars from the early sixties until the present day have chosen the scientific model of single brain studies.[1] This model has produced immensely valuable technology and exciting advances in knowledge of the study of a single mind/brain through the development of MRI (magnetic resonance imaging) and PET (positron emission tomography) scanning. But the experience of listening to music within the dynamic interchange within the consulting room is even more complex than the studies quoted above. This is partly because there are at least two brains/minds involved in this enterprise and these brains/minds are in dynamic mental communication with each other as well as being caught up in the experience of music, which is in dynamic motion within itself and in relation to each listener. I say 'at least' here because our brains/minds are also shaped by our ancestors, so that there is never a completely isolated brain/mind without continuing early relational and hereditary influence, even if this relation is avoidant.

As stated above, Judith Becker writing on 'Anthropological perspectives on music and emotion' addresses this context of listening to music in which there is more than one person involved. She challenges the single brain approach to studying the emotional experience of listening to music by holding the view that in reality there are more emotional experiences involved than that of the single listener. She writes:

> 'First-person descriptions of music and emotion are rife with interiority yet the understanding of how music affects interiors takes place within consensual, shared views of what makes up reality. Musical events set up an aural domain of co-ordination that envelops all those present.'[1]

Here Becker seems to be describing the consensual exterior shared views of what makes up reality. But what are these musical events that set up an aural domain of co-ordination that envelops all those present? One answer would be a choir, where there is a consensus that singing music is enjoyable and certainly co-ordination envelops all those present in the physical activity of singing together. Another event would be the pop concert where listening to the music and physically moving in a co-ordinated way with it would envelop all those present. Even listening to music alone is a consensual event in that the listener may allow themselves silently to share their view of what makes up reality with the composer or singer of the words/music of the song. But when there are no words, the feeling shapes or 'forms of feeling' which move the body in terms of emotion and blood pressure, etc. are communicated through tonal patterns by a composer and then further through a performer. The listener is in dynamic communication with another person's brain processes through the dynamic shapings in the music that are formed by the composer and further communicated by the performer.

Music within *word-based* psychotherapy is another such event which recognises the context of the human encounter between patient and therapist, but which could be said to focus more on interior right-brain communication as it becomes more verbal and engages more fully with the left brain. Becker describes such a context as a '*habitus*' of experiencing music which is:

> 'Complex systems of thought and behaviour concerning what music means, what it is for, how it is perceived and what might be appropriate expressive responses.'

But traditional music therapy is another such habitus of experiencing music. It is a consensual co-ordinated activity, which certainly envelops the therapist and the patient, and attention is rightly drawn to the exterior contexts of such an encounter alongside a recognition that there is movement within and between the brain/mind of therapist and patient.

Music therapy

What is music therapy and how does it connect with music within psychotherapy? According to Bunt and Pavlicevic:

> 'Music therapy is the use of sounds and music within an evolving relationship between child or adult and therapist to support and encourage physical, mental, social and emotional well-being.'[2]

This definition in a broad sense covers what is going on with the musical engagement within psychotherapy. However, what more can be said specifically about what is generally understood as music therapy?

According to Mercedes Pavlicevic and Leslie Bunt, music therapy has two main approaches, the *active* and the *receptive*. The active approach consists of joint musical improvisation between patient and therapist and 'Patients are encouraged to articulate their emotions externally by forming musical gestures and structures.' [2] The emphasis here could be said to be on the intermusical engagement over the interpersonal psychotherapeutic exchange.

In the receptive approach 'Various emotions can be aroused while listening to pre-composed music – played live by the therapist or on a recording'.[2] In the receptive approach described here it is not clear who chooses the music. Generally speaking, within the context of listening to music within *psychotherapy* it would seem appropriate for the patient to choose the music, given that the focus is on the growth of their inner sense of self-in-relationship; but there may be physical, mental and psychiatric states where this choice is not appropriate for the patient. There seems to be a grey area here depending on the context of the engagement.

In both the active and receptive modes, however, within traditional music therapy there are said to be:

> 'Very close connections in the chain of communication between the originator of the music and the recipient' and also 'overlapping links between music and emotions, therapeutic relationship, and the various needs of the patients'.[2]

This broad description of therapist/patient engagement in music therapy as described above has been developed over the last 50 years and is found in a variety of settings, such as pre-school centres and children's nurseries, special schools and units for children with learning difficulties; hospitals and special units for adults with learning difficulties, physical disabilities, mental health and neurological problems; hospital units and centres for older people and for people with visual or hearing impairments; hospices and special centres for people living with terminal illness and the prison and probation service.[2]

However, another form of music therapy created by Helen Bonny and practised worldwide is Guided Imagery and Music (GIM). This is described as follows:

> ' "Guided Imagery and Music" or "GIM" refers to all forms of music-imaging in an expanded state of consciousness, including not only the specific individual and group forms that Bonny developed, but also all variations and modifications in those forms created by her followers.'[3]

In this discipline the GIM practitioner *chooses* a programme of music to be listened to which is further tailored to the patient's needs. In other words, the patient might be asked whether one piece of music or another is more acceptable. Aspects of psychotherapy, such as transference and counter-transference, have been explored in the GIM process.[4] There has been on-going research and, for example, in one research study it was found that:

> 'GIM affects B-endorphine levels and in healthy subjects may lower depression levels. Unfortunately the sample size was too small to determine statistically significant results. The other study indicated that GIM appears

to lower depression and significantly increases the experience of a more meaningful and manageable life.'[5]

This patient group would seem to be more healthy psychologically than the music therapy patients described above by Bunt and Pavlicevic, who had a variety of disabilities and psychological problems which would exclude them from GIM. According to Cohen, these more severe cases include persons 'who lack sufficient ego strength and boundaries' and in such instances GIM might be 'a frightening and potentially harmful venture into the darker recesses of the self'.[6] Other persons who might not be suitable are those:

> 'who are acutely psychotic and those with dementia, persons in acute phases of substance withdrawal, or those without the necessary cognitive skills to interpret the abstract material from their unconscious'.[7]

Other receptive forms of music therapy from Germany which are of particular interest are the Resource-Oriented Music Therapy of Christoph Schwabe and Isabelle Frohne-Hagemann's Artistic Media and Music Therapy. There is also interesting research work being done by Lars Ole Bonde in Denmark. I will consider Christoph Schwabe's contribution to music therapy first. Even Rudd writes:

> 'Christoph Schwabe has maintained some basic human values, a concept of the individual, which reminds us that we are not only biological and individual creatures, but social beings as well.'[8]

This quotation would seem to resonate with the self-in-relation ideas put forward in this present book, in that not only is the person in the foreground rather than the music, but this person is an individual-in-relation to society rather than only an individual self.

Schwabe describes his work from 1996–2000 as a resource oriented psychotherapy, and he focuses on the healthy resources in patients and on rediscovering these resources in active and reflective listening, that is improvisation and listening. He writes of his treatment of patients in the psychiatric hospital, where 'sleeping therapy was the psychotherapeutic method of choice' and he felt that other methods which functioned as a 'wake up' on the one hand, and enabled self reflection on the other, should be attempted. He felt he needed to address the real conflict situations of the patients. He writes:

> 'The aims were no longer suggestion and relaxation but active confrontation and reflection. In this process music therapy led the way.'[9]

In these difficult conditions and with extremely ill patients he evolved 'Regulative Music Therapy'. This is a psychotherapy approach which 'aimed at furthering self-reflection by means of listening to music in a meditative setting'.[9] It is said to stimulate a:

> 'free non-intentional and accepting state of awareness floating between the awareness of music and the awareness of own emotions, thoughts and body

sensations . . . . Based on the diagnostic background conditions this per-
ceptive–psychological approach can on the one hand lead to direct confronta-
tion with partly conscious, and subconscious repressive mechanisms and,
thus, allow direct access to pathological limitations. On the other hand it can
stimulate the extension of awareness toward unused or underdeveloped
experiences'.[9]

This Regulative Music Therapy approach has been used in the psychotherapeutic treatment of psychosomatic in-patients and grew extensively in the
nineties in social day-care therapy and in the care of handicapped persons. With
such patients there is said to be the complicated and interesting issue of music
selection which unfortunately Schwabe does not discuss further.[9]

This Regulative Music Therapy approach has much in common with music
within individual psychotherapy, especially in the finding and support of the
self-in-relationship of the patient, but the main difference is that the therapist
in Schwabe's method seems to choose the music in the therapeutic work.

I turn now to the second theoretical approach to listening to music, which is
of particular interest. This is the thinking of Isabelle Frohne-Hagemann in her
paper 'Artistic media and music therapy'.[10] Her writing seems to resonate with
important theoretical strands underpinning music in word-based psychotherapy.

In her multi-medial approach to therapy she considers music, dance, painting
and poetry. Her thinking integrates music, movement, visual arts and poetry
and she sees these as belonging to the analogue mode of engaging with the
world. In contrast to this analogue way of perceiving the world there is the
discrete, digital or, as she writes, 'analytical' mode 'which relates things to each
other in a logical way'.[10]

Her thinking on this analogue mode is further underpinned by Zuckerkandl
and his writing on music as 'motion in the dynamic field of tones', which
identifies the dynamic movement of 'away from' and 'towards' in the motion of
the tones themselves in any piece of music, and especially within the musical
gestalt, that is, the fundamental 'whole form' of the diatonic scale.[11]

In Western society, music is rooted mostly in the diatonic scale (doh, re, me,
fah, soh, etc.). The tonic note, which is the first sounding tone of the scale, is in
musical relation to the dominant note, the fifth sounding tone. This interval of a
fifth is said to carry all the tonal relations of the scale and ultimately within the
tonic note itself.[11]

These musical relations occur because of the 'harmonic series', which are
mathematically related vibrations occurring naturally in sounding tones within
the diatonic scale. These vibrations occur in proportion, for example, they
double at the octave, and our ears 'hear' all the notes above and below as
multiples of the fundamental sounding tone or as halves or quarters. The
sounding tones of the diatonic scale are therefore closely related. Frohne-
Hagemann develops this thinking on the relational gestalt of the diatonic
scale linking these tonal relationships to the persons experiencing them. She
writes:

'This experience (relational gestalt) in the musical dimension of space and time also encompasses the *levels of relationship* between the individuals playing and singing.'[12]

In other words we are all caught up in a gestalt of tonal communication, that is, in a configuration of intense or less intense relationships in our playing or singing of music or listening to it. These relationships come alive as it were in our playing or singing. This idea of a musical gestalt being bound up with interpersonal relations appears again in the work of Trevarthen and Malloch.[13] Here an overlap is seen and heard to happen between the musical relationships of the diatonic scale and the infant/mother/carer relations observed in the musical/gestural and affective exchanges between them. This overlap of the dynamic musical relational analogue flow between music and persons-in-relationship is named as 'communicative musicality'. This communicative musicality will be discussed more fully in Chapter 9.

Another interesting aspect of Frohne-Hagemann's thinking is that she observes a hierarchy in the development of human physical senses in her mixed modal process of therapy. This hierarchy seems to follow the developmental progress of the growing infant-in-relationship. It begins with the infant in the womb where movement and hearing develop before the sense of sight and then speech. In the case study to be explored later in this book it is music which is first engaged with, then painting and then poetry. This process of early human development would seem to be mirrored in this case study.

In Denmark, Lars Ole Bonde is a current practitioner of BMGIM (the Bonny Method of Guided Imagery in Music) and works with cancer survivors. He is inspired by Ricoeur's theories of metaphor and narrative and has adapted Ricoeur's thinking to produce three specific experiential levels:

- the narrative episode
- the narrative configuration of the ego and the self
- the complete narrative.

He writes:

'Cancer rehabilitation is an important area within the healthcare system. After termination of medical treatment most cancer survivors have very few options for support, especially if they need psychological or psychosocial support.'[14]

Lars Ole Bonde's main research question is, 'What is the influence of ten individual BMGIM sessions on mood and quality of life in cancer survivors?'.

In the case study he addresses the more specific questions of, 'How does one cancer survivor experience the BMGIM process?'. He then asks, 'How does the imagery develop and/or how is it reconfigured during the ten BMGIM sessions?'.

In his work he has demonstrated, in the case study of Mrs J, that working with the BMGIM process has helped her develop new coping strategies to live her life more fully. He is currently involved in cancer care projects and in the development of an international network for research in music therapy and oncology. This important work uses metaphor and narrative in the patient's experience of listening to music. The music is chosen by the BMGIM therapist and not the patient. This would be an example of the informed choice of the therapist to assist recovery from serious physical illness that has a strong psychological impact. Of particular interest in this book is his question on how the imagery develops. This developing process is particularly noted in the case study of Liz in Chapter 10.

Differences and similarities in music used as a therapeutic medium

In terms of sameness, all four therapeutic receptive methods of GIM are concerned with the patient's emotional response, thinking and experience of listening to music. Apart from the receptive mode of listening to music, which is common to all four, there are three important basic differences.

The first is that, in listening to music within psychotherapy, the practice is centred in word-based psychotherapy and the practitioner would usually be a psychotherapist and not a music therapist. Because this is a different model of therapy and the approach itself is different, the music is chosen solely by the patient, as the therapist's choice would be understood as an intrusion and an imposition in this discipline. Apart from this, most psychotherapists are not trained musicians let alone trained in BMGIM or Regulative Music Therapy.

The second important difference is that in GIM the process is centred primarily in the music and many of the music therapists choose a prescriptive menu of music in agreement with the patient. The emphasis is on the music, the imagery and the 'journey', the purpose of which is healing, self development and spiritual growth.[15]

The third difference is that in GIM there does not seem to be an emphasis nor a focus on the sometimes intense relationship between the patient and therapist. In psychotherapy the importance of working through this interpersonal intensity to a more equable position for both of them is held to be an important stage in growing in relationship. Put briefly, music within psychotherapy, as presented in this book, is about a hoped-for growth in self-in-relationship for the patient and therapist, and in GIM the emphasis is about growth of self of the patient/client (which is different from self-in-relationship) although in GIM it is also about spiritual growth.

From a different perspective, Even Rudd writes on Schwabe's work with patients in a psychiatric hospital:

> 'Music is a kind of action in itself, creating the best possibilities for action leading towards rediscovery of our health resources. In these formulations Schwabe has planted the seed of a philosophy of music therapy with a social consciousness, which goes beyond the individual approach so often manifested in much thinking about therapy and treatment.'[8]

These are different models and aims of therapeutic practice, and music is used differently. In listening to music within psychotherapy, music is used *if* it comes into the room, whilst in BMGIM the whole structure of the therapeutic process is said to be focused in the music. Listening to music within psychotherapy is also aware of the dimension of social consciousness aimed for in Regulative Music Therapy. As has been said above, the patient chooses what music he or she wants to hear in listening to music within psychotherapy; also, the focus on being a self-in-relationship rather than an individual self contributes to the dimension of social consciousness.

The practice of listening to music within psychotherapy in action

In this form of listening to music therapeutically, the emphasis is on the interpersonal affective therapeutic communication between patient and therapist. The patient–therapist verbal exchange usually occurs at the end of the musical listening experience. The therapist listens to the meaning of the music for the patient and monitors the narrative emotional flow experienced by the patient and herself and observes the linkages between the patient's choice of music and the emotional and situational context of the work. These linkages (as will be noted in the case study material, *see* Chapter 10) seem to build into narratives of experienced sadness, anger, hope, joy, ambivalence, and acceptance of reality, all within the joint experience of listening to the passages of music.

There may not, however, be a verbal exchange between patient and therapist on the content of the music. The patient may be 'hiding' in a non-conscious attempt not to recall the inner trauma and pain which may have been too early to process in words, and music has become the safe protected hiding place to contain it. This would be a dissociative process but the effects may be felt in the patient's body and the body of the therapist, indicating this hidden trauma. This trauma may be further processed in a symbolic way through painting or drawing.

The therapist here must attend to the context of when the patient brought music into the room and then rely on right-brain-to-right-brain communication with them through listening to it together. This will involve being sensitive to the body movement, facial expression and vocal sounds of the patient, as well as realising that the therapist may be becoming what the music might be for the patient, that is, a safe protective container, but this time a personal container who is in relationship with the patient.

In Chapter 10, which describes the patient Liz's journey through the process of music within word-based psychotherapy, it is noted that Liz's initial choice of music to listen to was *The Dream of Gerontius*. This is the story of a soul's journey towards God, the ultimate container of being-in-relationship. The soul is protected on this journey by an angel who guards the soul and keeps it safe and temporally contains it on its journey towards God. There is strong symbolism here suggesting the hoped for safety of the therapeutic relationship on this healing journey.

When and if music comes into the room within psychotherapy, it is encountered as a medium in which the patient's inner experience is paramount, even though the therapist fully enters into the experience of the music herself. In fact the therapist will hold both experiences, that of the patient and her own, which will be noted in the background as it were. This relational position may well be a beginning of a growth process of self-in-relationship for the patient and the therapist. This depends on finding the developmental point of trauma, or in more severe cases, the early pre-verbal experience and unravelling together the developmental dissociation in the patient's life. This pre-verbal period is said to be from 0 until about 3 years of age. During this time, the left brain becomes more connected with the right brain and verbal language in individual words, phrases and sentences 'come on stream', as it were, for the infant. The infant is developing consciousness continually during this time.

Consciousness and the unconscious realm

This pre-conscious state is different from the 'unconscious', which is a Freudian description of the repressed deep areas of the psyche not generally available to conscious thought. The Jungian unconscious realm, however, is the shadow of consciousness. This shadow is said to come about through the growth of consciousness and not only through the forces of repression:

> 'Aside from what the personality represses while it organises itself and in addition to those things resulting from its choices, there exist dynamics that have not yet had a chance to become conscious.'[16]

This quotation could be said to describe the developing processes of the growing infant, child and adult.

There are two parts, therefore, to think about in listening to music in psychotherapy; one is witnessing the freeing up of what the patient has repressed and also taking note of the part of themselves which has not yet had a chance to grow. This will of course also require that the patient acknowledges the 'shadow side' of their psyche. The shadow side consists of the unacceptable (positive and negative) parts of ourselves which reside 'in the shadows', that area about which our ego is in the dark. Jung was very aware that music was a gateway to this realm of the dynamic unconscious.

New thinking on music and the unconscious

In conversation with Margaret Tilly about how she worked with patients in music therapy, Jung is reported as saying that music should be a part of every analysis. McGuire writes of this conversation:

'He (Jung) was very excited and as easy and naive as a child to work with. Finally he burst out with, "This opens up whole new avenues of research I'd never dreamed of. Because of what you've shown me this afternoon not just what you've said, but what I have actually felt and experienced – I feel that from now on music should be an essential part of every analysis. This reaches the deep archetypal material that we can only sometimes reach in our analytic work with patients. This is most remarkable."'[1]

This statement that music should be part of every analysis has certainly not been taken up by the analytic community, who have concentrated almost exclusively on verbal analysis. But Jung was particularly sensitive to music. He wrote:

'Music has certainly to do with the collective unconscious. This is evident in Wagner for example . . . Music expresses in sounds what fantasies and visions express in visual images. I am not a musician and would not be able to develop these ideas for you in detail. I can only draw your attention to the fact that music represents the movement, development and transformation of the motifs of the collective unconscious.'[18]

What Jung means by the 'collective unconscious' is the deepest layer within every human psyche. It is:

'the repository of all humankind's psychic heritage and possibilities. Just as our biological heritage is reflected in the growth and development of the human embryo, our psychic heritage is reflected in the collective unconscious, which is made up of archtypes.'[19]

These archetypes are common psychological patterns of behaviour, and it is how we structure these patterns of behaviour in our minds. For example, someone might appear as the wise old man or woman in our lives, or the 'Mother' figure, all loving, powerful, kind, etc. These are the motifs of the collective unconscious.

New writing in musicology is beginning to articulate more clearly the deep archetypal meanings of this world of sound and movement which is music. They are now in the twenty-first century engaged in the development of the ideas which Jung was referring to. The work of Victoria Adamenko on Jung and twentieth century music,[20] Byron Almen on 'Jung's Function-Attitudes in Music Composition and Discourse',[21] Robin Wallace on 'The Articulation of Gender in Brahms' *Third Symphony*: A Jungian View'[22] and Jeffrey Kurtzman on 'The Failure of Individuation in Monteverdi's *Orfeo*: The Psychic Disintegration of a Demigod'[23] are four examples of writing within musicology which reach outwards or inwards to the unconscious experience of listening to music.

The work of Austin Clarkson of York University, Toronto, Canada moves even nearer to exploring the unconscious experience of music. He focuses on applied Jungian theory and one course in particular, the 'Structures of Fantasy and Fantasies of Structures: Engaging the Aesthetic Self' is of special interest here.[24] He writes on the creative imagination in music and art in groups. This work on the creative imagination and aesthetic experience is the same inner territory occupied in the case study with Liz in Chapter 10.

This interest in Jungian ideas and musicology is an important move towards exploring personal experience in listening to music and can be seen as a further step towards accepting the experience and practice of listening to music chosen by the patient in verbal psychotherapy. A new language and discourse is being formulated within musicology which Jung himself would have welcomed.

But what do we now know about the practice of listening to music within psychotherapy? It is indeed related to verbal psychotherapy, music therapy, BMGIM and Regulative Music Therapy. It is not an isolated idea and it has drawn on the theory and practice of sociology, psychology, neuroscience, music therapy and now musicology. But the problem that is still central to this enquiry is: How might we begin to think about the linkage between music and interpersonal relationship? Is there any hard evidence here to support this idea that is the corner stone of this practice?

In the next chapter I will explore the origin of being a self-in-relationship and music. Trevarthen and Malloch's and Malloch's recent work on the infant–mother relationship and music will be some hard evidence and a central foundation from which to begin to answer these questions.[13,25] Panksepp's and Bernatzky's work on the experience of listening to music in an adult context will also be considered.[26] And, how the early relational pre-verbal musical relationship might be linked to the adult self-in-relationship within music in word-based psychotherapy will be introduced.

References

1 Becker J (2001) Anthropological perspectives on music and emotion. In: P Juslin and J Sloboda (eds) *Music and Emotion.* Oxford University Press, Oxford, p. 151.
2 Bunt L and Pavlicevic M (2001) Perspectives from music therapy. In: P Juslin and J Sloboda (eds) *Music and Emotion.* Oxford University Press, Oxford, p. 182.
3 Bruscia K and Grocke D (eds) (2002) *Guided Imagery and Music.* Barcelona Publications, Gilsum NH, p. xxi.
4 Bruschia K (1998) The dynamics of music psychotherapy. Quoted in: L Bruscia and D Grocke (eds) (2002) *Guided Imagery and Music.* Barcelona Publications, Gilsum NH, p. xxx.
5 Bruscia K and Grocke D (eds) (2002) *Guided Imagery and Music.* Barcelona Publications, Gilsum NH, p. xxxi.
6 Cohen N (2002) Ethical considerations in guided imagery and music. In L Bruscia and D Grocke (eds) *Guided Imagery and Music.* Barcelona Publications, Gilsum NH, p. 491.
7 Ibid, p. 492.
8 Rudd E (2005) Introduction to Christoph Schwabe: resource orientated music therapy. The development of a concept. *Nordic Journal of Music Therapy.* **14**(1): 48.
9 Ibid, p. 53.
10 Frohne-Hagemann I (2005) Artistic media and music therapy. *Nordic Journal of Music Therapy.* **14**(2): 168–78.

11 Zuckerkandl V (1956) *Sound and Symbol.* Princeton University Press, Princeton, NJ, pp. 228–33. (Reprinted 1973).

12 Frohne-Hagemann I (2005) Artistic media and music therapy. *Nordic Journal of Music Therapy.* **14**(2): 170.

13 Trevarthen C and Malloch S (2002) The musical lives of babies and families. *Journal of Zero to Three: National Center for Infants, Toddlers and Families.* **23**(1): 11.

14 Bonde LO (2005) 'Finding a New Place.' Metaphor and narrative in one cancer survivor's BMGIM therapy. *Nordic Journal of Music Therapy.* **14**(2): 137.

15 Bruscia K (2002) Preface: An opening metaphor. In: K Bruscia and D Grocke (eds) *Guided Imagery and Music.* Barcelona Publications, Gilsum NH, p. xxi.

16 Humbert E (1988) *CG Jung.* Chiron Publications, Illinois, pp. 48–9.

17 Ward KM (2002) A Jungian Orientation to the Bonny Method. In: K Bruscia and D Grocke (eds) *Guided Imagery in Music.* Barcelona Publications, Gilsum NH, p. 209.

18 Ibid, p. 210.

19 Ibid, p. 217.

20 Adamenko V (2006) *Jung and Twentieth-Century Music.* Proceedings of the International Association for Jungian Studies Conference 'Psyche and Imagination', University of Greenwich.

21 Almen B (2006) *Jung's Function-Attitudes in Music Composition and Discourse.* Proceedings of the International Association for Jungian Studies Conference 'Psyche and Imagination', University of Greenwich.

22 Wallace R (2006) *The Articulation of Gender in Brahms's 'Third Symphony': A Jungian View.* Proceedings of the International Association for Jungian Studies Conference 'Psyche and Imagination', University of Greenwich.

23 Kurtzman J (2006) *The Failure of Individuation in Monteverdi's Orfeo: The Psychic Disintegration of a Demigod.* Proceedings of the International Association for Jungian Studies Conference 'Psyche and Imagination', University of Greenwich.

24 Clarkson A (2006) 'Structures of Fantasy and Fantasies of Structures: Engaging the aesthetic self'. Unpublished paper.

25 Malloch S (1999) Mothers and infants and communicative musicality. *Musicae Scientiae.* (Special issue 1999–2000). The European Society for Cognitive Sciences, Belgium, pp. 21–31.

26 Panksepp J and Bernatzky G (2002) Emotional sounds and the brain: the neuro-affective foundations of musical appreciation. *Behavioural Processes.* **60**: 133–55.

CHAPTER 9

The experience of the origins of self-in-relationship in neuroscience and music

In the last chapter Becker described the 'habitus' of listening to music as a place of 'complex systems of thought and behaviour concerning what music means, what it is for, how it is to be perceived and what might be appropriate kinds of expressive responses'.[1]

But where might we begin to study this habitus of listening to music within psychotherapy? Because every client has been a baby and has had a primal carer, the work of Colwyn Trevarthen and Stephen Malloch on listening and making music within the infant–mother context might be a good place to start. Through their work we are now able to see, understand and measure what is going on between mother/carer and infant through their intimate gestures and lively loving movements. This work is centred on what is called 'communicative musicality' and we will consider this more fully.

We will then explore what it is to be a self and self-in-relationship within 'communicative musicality' and we will consider Panksepp's ideas on music and movement identified in the human substratas of the brain, which link Zuckerkandl's thinking on music and movement that he places at the dynamic core of life itself.

Communicative musicality

When a small infant gurgles with delight when his mother looks into his eyes and smiles, coos and moves towards him, there is an exchange of delight between them. This delight is expressed through their moving bodies and sounds, which carry the dynamic shapes of shared feeling.

Much research work has been done on such infant–mother interactions by, for example, Beebe *et al.*, Fogel and Thelen, Tronick and Weinberg.[2–4] However, although these researchers have often perceived the infant–mother or carers interactions to be musical, Stephen Malloch's work addresses the elements that go to make up what it is exactly that is musical about these interactions. He describes this kind of infant–mother or carer engagement as 'communicative musicality' and defines this as follows:

'Communicative musicality is the art of human companionable communication. It consists of our innate abilities, which function from birth, for being able to move sympathetically with another. It is the vehicle which carries emotion from one to another.'[5]

Trevarthen and Malloch write further that:

'The music-like relationship that we have seen between parent and infant reveals the raw materials that are utilised in music therapy.'[6]

However, it is my view that not only does this music-like relationship use the raw materials that are utilised in conventional music therapy, but communicative musicality can also be found in the practice of conventional word-based psychodynamic psychotherapy, where the body gestures and feeling tone are empathically engaged with and the process becomes music-like for a passage of time. It also lies at the heart of listening to music within psychotherapy for adults. This practice of listening to music within psychotherapy could be called *enhanced* communicative musicality because listening to music itself is involved.

Malloch and Trevarthen's concept of communicative musicality exists in the dynamic space between musical sounds and persons. It is not completely of musical sounds nor is it completely within the individual person. It is the overlap of two dynamic fields, that of musical sounds and that of persons-in-relationship, seen, felt and heard with their whole bodies. This will be explored more fully in Chapter 11.

However, from a neuroscientific perspective on adult responses to music, Panksepp and Bernatzky write:

'Well constructed music is uniquely efficacious in resonating with our basic emotional systems, bringing to life many affective proclivities that may be encoded, as birthrights, with ancient neural circuits constructed by our genes, many of which we share homologously with other mammals.'[7]

But what are these affective proclivities that may be encoded within our ancient neural circuits and which resonate with our basic emotional systems and are the raw materials that are utilised in music therapy?

The work of Trevarthen and Malloch could be said to have identified these affective proclivities. In Malloch's paper 'Mothers and infants and communicative musicality',[8] he has explored and examined mother–infant vocalisations using computer-based acoustic analysis. Both mother and baby are involved in vocal contours of sound, which can be quite brief or of longer duration. These were analysed in terms of pulse, quality and narrative in the infant–mother exchanges. Malloch and Trevarthen have found this communicative musicality to be the well-spring or source of the stories we tell one another of what we do and who we are in relationship. Along with Trevarthen, Malloch believes that:

'Narratives allow two persons to share a sense of passing time and to create and share the emotional envelopes that evolve through this shared time. They are said to be "the very essence of human companionship".'[8]

These stories or narratives we tell as adults of who we are in-relationship have their origin in the first narratives we experience as infants in relation to our mother or primary carer. Trevarthen and Schogler write:

'From the first "protoconversations" and in the earliest baby songs, meanings are made in emotional narratives, and forms of expression become habits that confirm the sharing of experiences over time. They become part of the history of companionship, first in intimate family relationships, then in the daily work of the wider community.'[9]

However, from the beginning these narratives are built from units of pulse and quality found in the jointly created gestures of vocalisations and bodily movement. They enliven us. They make life interesting. But let us examine in more detail what we mean by pulse and quality, which go to make these narratives.

Pulse

Musical pulse is defined as 'The regular succession of discrete behavioural steps through time, linking the present to the past, representing the "future creating" process by which a subject may anticipate what might happen and when'[10]and again pulse is 'The regular succession of discrete events through time, which we use to anticipate what might happen and when'.[6]

There is a regularity in pulse which builds into a sense of continuity or narrative for the infant which, according to Trevarthen, is the shape of effort, excitement, satisfaction and repose. When the regularity ceases at the end of the musical game there is a recognised kind of ending with the carer, a shared look or clap of the hands, and the end is noted but the friendship and companionship continues. It is only an ending within the continuing relationship, not *the* end of the relationship. The repeated experience of regular pulse through time through shared music is an early shared adventure for the infant in that some joyful episodes in time do end but they can look forward with hope to them starting again. When the baby is engaged with the experience of regular sharing of pulse in a musical game or song with a carer, they experience the passing of time, shared time in single steps and emotive sequences with a companion.

Davis and Wallbridge quote Winnicott on the importance of this sense of continuity in time in the day-to-day caring experience of the mother with the child and refer to it as 'the benign sequence'. They write:

'The sense of continuous time in the infant comes to be added through the completion of *processes* – processes which from the outside may seem to be purely physiological but which belong to infant psychology and take place in a complex psychological field, determined by the awareness of empathy of the mother.'[11]

But how exactly is this sympathy communicated? In the mother–child vocal/ musical engagement, shared contours of sound in which the mother or carer first imitates and then elaborates the melodic line could be said to communicate the empathic feeling tone and describe the *quality* of the mother/carer engagement with the infant. Lively melodic leaps of joy or gentle falling phrases carry the feeling tone along with matching hand or arm gestures.

Quality

Trevarthen and Malloch write on this element of quality. They describe it as movements and shared vocal contours, which present the quality of empathic communication. Quality in this context refers to 'the contours of expression moving through time',[10] and again 'Quality consists of the contours of expressive vocal and body gesture shaping time with expressive movements.'[10]

But how might these contours of changing expression in sound contribute to the quality of the expression? Trevarthen and Malloch write that in an attentive loving exchange, a parent will listen very attentively to the pitch, contour, tone timbre and harmony or dissonance of the child's vocalisation and will usually respond appropriately.[6] The parent may imitate directly the pitch contour of the infant, in other words a climbing, exuberant, sudden melodic phrase exclaimed by the baby will be immediately imitated precisely by the carer or with variations. Or the parent may do the opposite and respond with a contrasting melodic contour. In a 'good enough' infant–mother relationship there will be a balance of imitation and contrast. The timbre of the mother's or carer's voice, its sharpness, roughness contribute to the quality of the exchange. The mother and infant will be closely attentive to one another and move together in shared time through the different phases of expression. Agreeing with the research of Papousek and Papousek[12] and Trehub[13] and he himself observing the infant, Trevarthen and Schogler write:

> 'Their selective orientation to musical sounds, critical discrimination of musical features of sound, and vocal and gestural responses that are timed and expressed to contribute to a joint musical game, confirm that music has roots in human nature.'[14]

In a less than 'good enough' attunement exchange, which can occur in a mother suffering from post-natal depression, or where there are sensory or motor disorders of the infant, both parties will·suffer. Malloch[15] writes that in perturbation experiments carried out by Murray and Trevarthen[16] and Tronick *et al.*[17] when the mother was asked to keep a still face and remain silent in front of her infant for one minute, the baby protested. Malloch writes further that the infant seeks not only encouraging communicative forms of signal from its mother – the signals must be appropriately timed and inflected – it is vital that the infant receives vocal and gestural responses that fit with his or her innate predisposition to interact with another. We will now turn to narrative, the third element of communicative musicality.

Narrative

Trevarthen and Malloch write that the sequence of pulse and quality combine to form vocal narratives of shared emotion and experience and through these narratives they sustain a co-ordinated relationship through time.[10]

In the whole spectrum of gestural motion of shared musical sounds, when mother and infant are engaged in shared time in music, shared emotional narratives are engaged in. In such a musical game a sense of self-in-relation and continuity in terms of time and process are being built up for both of them. Malloch writes that:

> 'Narratives of individual experience and of companionship are built from the units of pulse and quality found in the jointly created gestures of vocalisations and bodily movement. Narratives are the very essence of human companionship and communication. Narration allows two persons to share a sense of passing time, and to create and share a particular experience in relation which evolves through this shared time.'[8]

This means that the infant experiences the story of themself-in-relation to the carer. Through musical narrative, the meaning of who they are in-relationship is born out of this communicative musicality.

This could also describe something of what happens to the client's self-in-relationship within listening to music in psychotherapy. The clients' narrative of who they were and are in relationship slowly evolves through the rhythm, pulse, melody and harmony of the shared 'communicative musicality' in the therapeutic relationship. The added shared experience of listening to music enhances this process of therapeutic 'communicative musicality'. We will explore this therapeutic musical experience in the consulting room more fully in Chapter 11.

So far we have shown how musical sounds are intrinsically bound up with becoming more of a baby-in-relationship with a primal carer. We have discussed communicative musicality which describes the ways in which the infant moves, makes musical sounds and corresponding gestures to indicate their motive for connection with the caring adult. But what do we know about the origins of this sense of self and self-in-relation?

The self and the self-in-relationship

Trevarthen writes that:

> 'The baby has a well-integrated self at birth, an effective self. But it has to work out what it has to do with this motivated life it has, and one of the first things it has to learn is the meaning of the world.'[18]

It would seem that human infant meaning begins to be fathomed in communication with a sympathetic adult. He writes further that 'There is no such thing as meaning found by a single self. Meaning has to be communicated and communicable.'[19]

Here Trevarthen is writing about the human infant developing within the relational gestalt of the family or other relational combination. In other words, a self-in-relation.

In the discipline of neuroscience, in which there is investigation of the infant brain before birth, the language is that of embryos, developing neural pathways, cerebral cortex, etc. and this needs to be so. However, Trevarthen writes that many of the structures that are going to be important in early communication are functioning in the brain long before the cerebral cortex is even beginning to be formed.[20] In the foetal stage the cortex is there, but very immature. The infant at this stage is starting to have an auditory awareness of other persons (or just the mother) as another. Here we are thinking mainly of musical sounds and the mother's voice that enter the space where the foetus may be listening. Trevarthen's view is supported by Mechthild Papousek, who writes that:

> 'The human newborn enters the extra-uterine environment with amazing predispositions to perceive, process and memorise music in its basic elements. External sounds and music and the more intimate sensations of the mother's speaking or singing voice already reach the foetus' inner ear 3 to 4 months prior to birth, contributing to the structural and functional maturation of central auditory pathways. The natural perceptual world of the foetus is enriched even earlier with bodily sensations of various vital rhythms produced by the mother's breathing, speaking, walking and dancing.'[21]

Here one is reminded of Zuckerkandl's thinking when he places music at the dynamic core of life itself.

What is being described above are human relational connections with the mother's body and her sounds at this time. But these *connections* are not generally highlighted. Before birth the embryo is in a womb from the start of existence and the womb is in a person, the 'habitus' of mother; a relational gestalt. This point having been made, we will turn to the world of neuroscience for the origin of the self-system of the infant within the mother's womb, remembering that this self-system is also a self-in-relationship.

The brain-in-relationship: the mind

Writing on art and neuro-psychoanalysis, Oppenheim states that neuroscientists such as Damasio and Panksepp would agree that the basic awareness for the human infant originates and emanates from subcortical core structures at the top of the brainstem.[22] Panksepp, in particular, posits an archaic 'primary template' of the SELF-system in the 'PAG', that is the 'primary circuits of the grey matter of the brainstem, the periaqueductal gray'. He writes that this SELF-schema may trigger bodily orientation. In other words, a way of being. This way of being is said to encourage the drawing out of values from the interaction of the inner milieu with outer stimuli. He states:

> 'This postulated SELF-schema presumably can trigger basic forms of bodily orientation and promote the extraction of values from the interaction of the internal milieu with environmental incentive stimuli.'[23]

Panksepp understands the PAG as an 'intrinsically dynamic substrata of consciousness', a kind of spontaneously active 'stage manager', that helps create a neuropsychic focus of existence. This neuro-psychic focus is said to provide an active platform for the emergence of 'higher observers' or later platforms that emerge as the SELF-process 'migrates' through higher regions of the brain.

This thinking would seem to resonate with that of Trevarthen in terms of the infant in the womb actively reaching out to new ways of being and being-in-relationship with mother and the outside world.

Trevarthen's infant, however, is motivated rhythmically with an Intrinsic Motive Formation (IMF) and an Intrinsic Motive Pulse (IMP). The IMF is a 'body imaging core system formed in the brain of a human embryo . . . It acts as a co-ordinator and regulator of movements and their prospective sensory control.' It also 'contains generators of neural time and dynamic tension'.[24] The IMP is 'the body-moving rhythmic and emotionally modulated system. Musicality is the aurally appreciated expression of the activity of the IMF with the IMP as its agent'.[25] Trevarthen's infant is motivated rhythmically with an IMF and an IMP.

The motivation of Trevarthen's human infant reminds us that Panksepp's neurobiological SELF-schema is still in attachment to mother as the infant grows in the womb. It is as the baby emerges and grows outside the womb and begins to be seen and heard to be in attachment or avoidant of attachment that a sense of self-in-relationship is generally observed.

In this attachment behaviour Panksepp's sense of SELF-schema triggers bodily orientation towards mother through mother's voice (which the infant has heard in the womb), her touch, and the sight of her face. It is at this stage of being born that Trevarthen's and Malloch's work on proto-conversation through music, that is, communicative musicality, is understood even more clearly.

Of course it is not a fully developed emotional, cognitive, reflective self-in-relationship at this stage. A growing sense of self-in-relationship may be observed throughout childhood generally reaching a fuller state of self-in-relationship towards adolescence or during adolescence, when the emerging adult is able to reflect more fully upon who they are and are becoming and have been. But there is a suggestion here that this primal sense of self-in-relationship and the emotions and intentional behaviour involved may be glimpsed in moments of shared time with an infant soon after birth. Trevarthen describes the observation of a 20-minute-old baby in India tracking the movement of a red ball on a string which is held by a visitor. He writes:

'The baby's attention is focused on a red ball that is being held by a nurse. The baby is tracking the ball with its nose, its mouth, its hands and its feet, and as the ball is moving around, the baby's body is pulled with it as a completely whole intentional agent. There is no question of this being a loosely connected bundle of reflexes. The baby is alive with a one-time, one-space mind.'[26]

He writes further of the nurse's involvement:

'They are playing a game together. This little person, 20-minutes-old, is involved in a game with an adult, demonstrating coherence of its intentionality and its awareness of a world outside the body, and especially a world that offers live company.'[26]

What has this to do with music in adult psychotherapy?

Music within psychotherapy attempts to explore not the self of the single brain structures of the client but the sense of self-in-relationship for the client. This is done through the engagement with music when a passage of music that the client chooses and needs to hear is brought into the consulting room. The sense of self-in-relationship that the client has experienced with significant others in the past is explored through the medium of music. The music, chosen by the client, is understood as enhancing and focusing on the particular relational brain configurations with significant others from the client's past.

Writing on the power of music to promote emotional health, Panksepp and Bekkedal write that music's power to evoke deep feelings and enliven emotions in the therapeutic context of restoring and sustaining health is much appreciated in emerging disciplines. But they also write that there is much uncertainty as to how effective it really is because as yet we don't know enough about how these effects are mediated within the enormous complexity of the brain. One possibility that is considered is that the beneficial effects are achieved 'via the ability of music to directly modify the neural substrates of affective states, which can then have widespread effects on the autonomic hormonal and immunologial mechanisms of the body'.[27]

In other words music reaches very deep into the substrata of the brain, where thinking strategies are not directly available but deep feeling or sensation states, such as love, sorrow etc., are. Following on from this, Panksepp and Bernatzky write that:

'Music derives its affective charge directly from dynamic aspects of brain systems that normally control real emotions and which are distinct from, albeit highly interactive with, cognitive processes.'[28]

This statement addresses the fact that many people appreciate music through their cognitive abilities, their capacity to think and reflect about it. But there is also something else going on, especially when some music is felt to be really important for us. Something else happens when we have strong emotional responses to music. Referring to research by Blood and Zatorre,[29] Panksepp and Bernatzky assert that, 'When music truly moves us, something quite dramatic happens in deep subcortical regions of our brains.'[7]

Panksepp and Bekkedal also comment on the habitus or context of any research on listening to music. Writing particularly on research into the happy and sad effects of music, they state that:

> 'First, to obtain powerful emotional effects, it will probably be important to allow listeners to choose the pieces of music which move them personally. To do otherwise is to compromise the intensity of affective experience for the benefit of experimental control, and that does not seem to be a reasonable initial choice from the vantage of clarifying how emotions in music modify cerebral processing.'[27]

This is an important recommendation because they clearly understand that the particular person's response to listening to a passage of music is his or her inner self-in-relationship and that this might be the real object of such research. It is the listener's individual experience of self-in-relationship, the neural connections that arise from these deep subcortical structures, which are being engaged within the experience of listening to music, which is important for us. This process therefore is unique for the individual and arises from the earliest adventures, journeys of discovery or stories made together, which are the 'communicative musicality' with our primary carers.

Listening to music in the consulting room

In the context or 'habitus' of listening to music in psychotherapy, the music that the patient needs to hear is brought into the room. Generally it is understood that, in psychodynamic psychotherapy, the feelings that the patient brings into the room may arise from early childhood experience, and it is the same understanding when the patient brings music into the room within word-based psychotherapy. But, as has been written above, the adult brain is incredibly complex and as yet there is uncertainty as to how music is processed for the given individual. But having found that music can be responded to very early in life and it has its roots in a fundamental substratum of the brain, the PAG, we must listen to this music in the consulting room, which may be evoking, through its shapes of feeling, the deep longings and needs of the patient from early in life, especially if these deep longings and needs seem to be non-verbal. But care must be taken here, for the feelings of hurt and loss brought into the consulting room may be secondary emotions not closely related to the prototypic state of 'separation distress'. This is where focused attention to the patient's history is important. The very early experience of separation distress is indicated where words to describe it are consistently unavailable for the patient.[30]

However, in this prototypic state, this place before words, the patient may come alive to the sound of emotionally significant music. In Liz's case, described in Chapter 10, her chosen music evoked a kind of being-in-relationship, a 'communicative musicality', which reached deeply or back non-verbally to a time before words were available, but where separation distress and also love and contentment were experienced in infancy.

Introducing Liz

Liz was separated from her mother at the age of six weeks when her grandmother began to look after her. When her mother felt a bit better, perhaps after some months, Liz was returned to her mother, who remained physically and emotionally fragile for many years.

It is interesting that the first music that Liz brought into the consulting room was that sung by the Angel in Elgar's *Dream of Gerontius* as she bears Gerontius' soul to God. The feelings of bitter-sweet sadness mingled with the soothing comforting of fear would be something sad to remember of what her grandmother's feeling state might have been as she began to care for this tiny baby of six weeks old. This experience of grandmother would have been felt by this tiny baby and this experience may have laid down connections in her early brain/mind.

Liz survived this first loss of her mother because of her grandmother whom she then 'lost' when Liz was returned to mother. Her mother, however, was in poor health and unable to attend to Liz's emotional needs She then lost her grandmother completely when she died when Liz was 11 years old. She could be said to have experienced a complex and traumatic series of losses by this early age and no one seemed to recognise this at this time. These feelings got buried only to re-emerge after the death of her father when Liz began therapy in 1992 with her first therapist. The history of her therapeutic engagement will be taken up more fully in Chapter 10.

Returning to music in the consulting room and following on from the *Dream of Gerontius*, Liz brought in a series of pieces of music which for a time dipped into this early relational way of being, this early 'communicative musicality', where it felt in the counter-transference that I was holding a very vulnerable and emotionally fragile bit of Liz's inner world. At times of holidays and breaks from therapy Liz would need to revisit the Angel passage from the *Dream of Gerontius* when she returned to therapy, before moving on to other pieces of music. These later pieces of music, these configurations of enhanced 'communicative musicality', could be thought of as other musical dynamic memories. The Angel passage, this myth or legend, might be described as resonating with the earliest source of 'communicative musicality', a bitter-sweet experience etched in the configurations of Liz's brain/mind.

How do we begin to think of the feelings of separation distress of the infant, which Liz was, and the feelings of wholeness, comfort and love she experienced through listening to music as an adult? In psychoanalytic language, Liz might have been experiencing me, the therapist, in the therapeutic transference as her early primal experience of the warm, supportive mother (whom she 'lost') and also her grandmother and her father. But how do we link the separation distress and the feelings of warmth and comfort?

Panksepp writes that these very different sensations are brought together in certain types of music, which provoke chills and have a bitter-sweet quality about them. He writes:

> 'In music that provokes chills, the wistful sense of loss and the possibility of reunion are profoundly blended in the dynamics of sound ... This audio-vocal experience speaks to us of our humanness and our profound relatedness to other people and the rest of nature.'[31]

What is really important here is that these early sensations or feelings of distress and comfort and love are blended in music. It is not distress *or* comfort, it is both. This echoes Langer's thinking that music can convey more than one sensation or feeling at the same time.[32] For the person who is drawn to this kind of music, the sorrow expressed is shot through with sensations or feelings of comforting joy. These complex feelings are carried for the patient or listener in the chosen piece of music and the feelings have to be worked through with the therapist or listener in the consulting room. How can this be better understood and how is it done?

To understand the process better we need to consider the child in the adult who is distressed within the infant–mother context. Here we would be describing a relational communicative gestalt where the intensities of sorrow and joy flow swiftly through each other and perhaps overlap. They would reach a special intensity when mother or appropriate carer would not have been readily available to soothe and help regulate the distress. In therapy, this special intensity would be seen and experienced around breaks in therapy.

In early life, if this distress and loss had gone on for too long, unassuaged by the presence of a comforting other, perhaps, for instance, in very difficult circumstances of a mother's illness, this experience of too much fear and anxiety would become etched in the infant's brain. These feelings may then become dissociated from everyday life and found again more safely in music. This child, when grown up, may seek out music with just this relational gestalt to convince her that the anxiety and fear of loss and the bliss of joy on reunion are connected in human experience. It could be a stored 'image' response in the right brain, before the verbal connections to the left brain come on stream as it were. This relational musical gestalt becomes *a parable* of the temporary 'good enough' mother/child relationship, a relationship which, through no-one's fault, was lost but hidden within music.[33] The aim of enhanced music psychotherapy would be to bring these painful bitter-sweet experiences into words and into the consulting room where they can be felt, first through communicative musicality as a way of being together, and then into words. It would seem that this happened to some degree as Liz became able to use words to write of her experience in poetry and then write episodes of her autobiography past and present.

When the adult person's life circumstances again evoke such feelings of love, loss and despair, listening or performing music alone may not be enough to regulate this early right-brain experiential pattern sufficiently. It may be appropriate that psychotherapy, a human receptive, self-regulating therapeutic relationship of enhanced communicative musicality is also engaged in.

Through transference and counter-transference, where not only the feelings are reflected in the chosen music, but a space for thinking about the context of these feelings is provided, there may be the start of the hoped for healing and re-ordering of the early neural pathways and the recognition and start of integration of the early experience of both loss and love. The undoing of the early relational trauma, the realisation that 'that happened then' and is 'not happening now' would be a powerful therapeutic place to have reached. This undoing process described by Wilkinson[34] will be considered more closely in Chapter 11.

References

1 Becker J (2001) Anthropological perspectives on music and emotion. In: P Juslin and J Sloboda (eds) *Music and Emotion*. Oxford University Press, Oxford, p. 151.

2 Beebe B, Stern D and Jaffe J (1979) The kinesic rhythm of mother–infant interactions. In: AW Siegman and S Feldstein (eds) *Of Speech and Time: temporal speech patterns in interpersonal contexts*. Erlbaum, Hillsdale, NJ.

3 Fogel A and Thelen E (1987) Development of early expressive action from a dynamic systems approach. *Developmental Psychology*. **23:** 747–61.

4 Tronick EZ and Weinberg MK (1997) Depressed mothers and infants: failure to form dyadic states of consciousness. In: L Murray and PJ Cooper (eds) *Postpartum Depression and Child Development*. Guildford Press, New York, pp. 54–81.

5 Malloch S (1999) Mothers and infants and communicative musicality. *Musicae Scientia. (Special issue 1999–2000)*. The European Society for Cognitive Sciences, Belgium, pp. 29–57.

6 Trevarthen C and Malloch S (2000) The dance of well being: the nature of the musical therapeutic effect. *The Norwegian Journal of Music Therapy*. **9**(2): 3–17.

7 Panksepp J and Bernatzky G (2002) Emotional sounds and the brain: the neuro-affective foundations of musical appreciation. *Behavioural Processes*. **60:** 133–55.

8 Malloch S (1999) Mothers and infants and communicative musicality. *Musicae Scientia. (Special issue 1999–2000)*. The European Society for Cognitive Sciences, Belgium, p. 45.

9 Trevarthen C and Schogler B (2005) Musicality and the creation of meaning: infant's voices and jazz duets show us how, not what music means. In: Cynthia M Grund (ed.) *Cross Disciplinary Studies in Music and Meaning*. Indiana University Press, Bloomington, Indianapolis, p. 17.

10 Trevarthen C and Malloch S (2002) The musical lives of babies and families. *Journal of Zero to Three*. National Centre for Infants, Toddlers and Families. **23**(1): 11.

11 Davis M and Wallbridge D (1990) *Boundary and Space: An introduction to the work of DW Winnicott*. Karnac Books Ltd., London, p. 170.

12 Papousek M and Papousek H (1981) Musical elements in the infant's vocalization: their significance for communication, cognition and creativity. In: LP Lipsitt and CK

Rovee-Corvier (eds) *Advances in Infancy Research* Vol.1. Ablex, Norwood, NJ, pp. 163–224.

13 Trehub SE (1990) The perception of musical patterns by human infants: the provision of similar patterns by their parents. In: MA Berkley and WC Stebbins (eds) *Comparative Perception* Vol.1 Mechanisms. Wiley, New York, pp. 429–59.

14 Trevarthen C and Schogler B (2005) Musicality and the creation of meaning: infant's voices and jazz duets show us how, not what, music means. In: Cynthia M. Grund (ed.) *Cross Disciplinary Studies in Music and Meaning*. Indiana University Press, Bloomington, Indianapolis.

15 Malloch S (1999) Mothers and infants and communicative musicality. *Musicae Scientiae*. Special Issue (1999–2000). The European Society for Cognitive Sciences, Belgium, pp. 21–31.

16 Murray L and Trevarthen C (1985) Emotional regulation of interactions between two-month-olds and their mothers. In: T Field and N Fox (eds) *Social Perception in Infants*. Albex, Norwood, NJ, pp. 177–97.

17 Tronick EZ *et al.* (1980) Monodic phases: a structural descriptive analysis of infant–mother face-to-face interaction. *Merril–Palmer Quarterly of Behaviour and Development.* **26:** 124.

18 Trevarthen C (2003) Neuroscience and intrinsic psychodynamics: current knowledge and potential for therapy. In: J Corrigal and H Wilkinson (eds) *Revolutionary Connections*. Karnac (Books) Ltd., London, p. 21.

19 Ibid, p. 67.

20 Ibid, p. 24.

21 Papousek M (2004) Foreword. In: M Nocker-Ribaupierre (ed.) *Music Therapy for Premature and Newborn Infants*. Barcelona Publishers, Gilsum.

22 Oppenheim L (2005) *A Curious Intimacy: art and neuro-psychoanalysis*. Routledge, London, p. 52.

23 Panksepp J (1998) *Affective Neuroscience: the foundations of human and animal emotions*. Oxford University Press, Oxford, p. 313.

24 Trevarthen C (1999) Musicality and the intrinsic motive pulse: evidence from human psychobiology and infant communication. *Musicae Scientiae*. Special Issue (1999–2000). The European Society for Cognitive Sciences, Belgium, p. 155.

25 Trevarthen C (2003) Neuroscience and intrinsic psychodynamics: current knowledge and potential for therapy. In: J Corrigall and H Wilkinson (eds) *Revolutionary Connections*. Karnac Books Ltd., London, pp. 56–7.

26 Ibid, p. 160.

27 Panksepp J and Bekkedal YV (1997) The affective cerebral consequence of music: happy vs sad effects of the EEG and clinical implications. *International Journal of Arts-Medicine*. **5**(1): 18–27.

28 Panksepp J and Bernatzky G (2002) Emotional sounds and the brain: the neuro-affective foundations of musical appreciation. *Behavioural Processes*. **60:** 135.

29 Blood AJ and Zatorre RJ (2001) Intensely pleasurable responses to music correlate with activity in brain regions implicated in reward and emotion. *Proceedings of the National Academy of Sciences*. **98:** 11818–23.

30 Watt DF (2003) Psychotherapy in an age of neuroscience: bridges to affective neuroscience. In: J Corrigall and H Wilkinson (eds) *Revolutionary Connections*. Karnac Books Ltd., London, pp. 88–9.

31 Panksepp J (1998) *Affective Neuroscience: the foundations of human and animal emotions*. Oxford University Press, Oxford, p. 279.

32 Langer SK (1942) *Philosophy in a New Key.* Harvard University Press, Cambridge, Mass. and London, p. 238. (Reprinted 1996).

33 Trevarthen C (2006) Wer schreibt die Autobiographie eines Kindes. Warum Menschen Sich Erinnern Können. (Fortschritte der Interdisziplinären Gedächtnisforschung) Hrsg. Hans Markowitsch und Harald Weltzer. Klett-Cotta, Stuttgart, pp. 225–55. (Translation: Karoline Tschuggnall).

34 Wilkinson M (2006) *Coming into Mind.* Routledge, East Sussex and New York.

PART 3

The Experience of Listening to Music within Psychotherapy

CHAPTER 10

A two-part invention

This chapter is a clinical example of listening to music chosen by the patient in word-based psychotherapy. My commentary is interspersed with Liz's written reflections. The chapter will describe some of the significant therapeutic work done with Liz on her return to therapy after six months.

Liz had worked in therapy since 1992, initially for four years with another therapist, who decided to refer her to me because she knew of my interest in music and knew that Liz was musical. Liz arrived in 1995 and after an initial attempt to work within joint music improvisation we moved on to the more usual word-based therapy. At this stage Liz seemed more able to articulate her mental pain. This phase of the work continued until 2002. In 2003 after a six-month break and having been diagnosed with fibromyalgia, Liz returned to therapy and we engaged in listening to music together, alongside verbal psychotherapy.

Active musical improvisation

When Liz first came into therapy with me in 1995, we explored ways of engaging through the practice of joint musical improvisation, which is the usual method associated with traditional music therapy. This involved Liz and myself sitting at the piano keyboard and playing together in the pentatonic scale. (This is to be found on the black notes of the piano.) The felt sensation of playing together in this way is of being caught up in a seamless holding sequence of sounds. The main musical sensation is the absence of overt dynamic tension between the sounds. I chose to work within the pentatonic scale because there would be no points of tension between our playing together, nothing which might jar her sense of being held securely.

Liz stayed in therapy with me from 1995 until December 2002. The description of the work described below will be from June 2003 until July 2004, during which time she returned to therapy to work within the context of listening to music with me.

The work will be presented on two levels. On the first level I will describe some of the content and the process of the therapy sessions. On the second level Liz will tell her story through her experiences of music, both singing and listening. It will be a kind of contrapuntal exercise; a two-part invention involving an account of the uneven ups and downs of the process of therapy alongside Liz's meta-narrative of how her chosen music is intertwined as a therapeutic medium in which we were both involved. We will begin with Liz's arrival in the room after a six-month break.

Initial return to therapy

Liz arrived carrying a walking stick. She was in pain and moved with difficulty. She had been attending a pain clinic. Because her physical symptoms and illness were known to me and brought into the room, as it were, I opened each session by asking directly how she was. It was usually quite a direct question regarding her health. It could be 'How are you Liz?'. This would cover how she wanted to answer. She could reply by talking about her physical symptoms and/or how she was feeling emotionally. This kind of question was different from the way I usually start a psychodynamic psychotherapy session. I usually wait for the patient to begin and give them space but in Liz's case and where there is physical illness involved I tend to begin by letting the client know by the above question that I care and am concerned about their physical health. It functions as an immediate psychological holding. It also provides a framework for feelings of closeness between the client and therapist and therapist and client. But if the client is not feeling well I need to attend to this obvious physical distress first.

On this initial session after a six-months' break, and after finding a comfortable sitting position, I asked 'How are you Liz?'. She described the physical pain in her limbs and the difficulties in following the instructions on exercises she had been prescribed by the pain clinic. She felt that a lot of the pain was associated with her mother. (Her mother had been in severe physical pain in her limbs for most of her life and Liz's childhood was lived in this shadow.) She said that she wanted to do some work on this. Because we had done many years of verbal psychodynamic work and had made significant progress in her sense of who she was in the world, I offered the possibility of listening to music of Liz's choice, together with thinking, talking and writing about it. This process might address now what might have been non-verbal and not ready to be engaged with earlier. It could also consolidate the work already achieved by deliberately having Liz write about what was happening for her. This perhaps would build on any new neural pathways and connections between the right-brain and the left-brain which had already begun in the earlier work. I talked to Liz about this and she agreed to try it.

For her first piece of music Liz chose *The Dream of Gerontius*, an oratorio by Elgar. In particular we focused on the passage about the angel gently leading Gerontius' soul to God on his death. The text of the oratorio is a poem by Cardinal John Henry Newman on the death of Gerontius and the story of his soul's journey to meet God. We decided to talk about this at the next session and she offered to bring in her CD. I already owned a CD of *The Dream of Gerontius* so I was also able to listen to it before we next met. The symbolism associated with her first choice of music is interesting. In the transference, I could be the embodied 'angel' leading Liz's inner self-in-relation on a painful journey which, in the end, would mean a richer kind of freedom for her.

We then talked about Handel's *Messiah* and the great Amen chorus and how these are also very powerful Christian narratives for her. Liz's strong faith in God is also evident here. It is the Messiah who comes with salvation and responded to by the angelic affirmation, 'Amen'. In a sung performance this angelic affirmation is also a sung human affirmation, 'Amen' meaning 'so be it'.

One could say that there are two psychological themes outlined by the chosen music. They are death and resurrection, and hopeless despair and the feeling of being saved.

Liz's reflection on beginning therapy

I first went to see Mary in June 1995. I had been referred to a previous therapist who had worked with me for four years. She realised that I had encountered a 'block' and thought that as I was a musical person, music in some form might unlock and make available painful feelings that I might be able to fully experience and name. Words were not always available to me and we hoped that sounds would help me begin to process any material that surfaced.

At first in 1995 Mary encouraged me to play the piano with her on the black notes using the pentatonic scale. We also played some percussion instruments. At the time I did not understand what was happening and was not sure that I would gain any benefit from this. But I carried on and found what felt like some kind of grief was being released and little by little I began talking again with Mary about my life at the time, my family and some of my early life as a child. The talking continued until December 2002.

Things were fine until the summer of 2003 when I was diagnosed with fibromyalgia and the specialist recommended an eight-week course of two days a week at a local unit attached to the hospital. This was a pain control programme that dealt with all aspects of pain and was designed to help me cope with the pain but not to find a cure. The course included education, discussions on pacing and activity movements and exercise sessions, an activity workshop and goal-setting sessions. There were sessions on 'What is stress?' and how to handle it. All of this I couldn't cope with.

I had previously talked with Mary about all aspects of my childhood, or so I had thought, but this bad experience in the pain clinic may have worked as a trigger to make accessible all sorts of material that I had been unable to reach before. When I explained all this to Mary she suggested that we went back to music to see if this might help me find words to express how I felt. We resumed our work together in the summer of 2003.

Liz's reflection on returning to therapy

We started by discussing how I listen to music and what affects me. As I have been a choral singer for the past twenty years, and before that would join anything so I could sing on a regular basis, along with lots of singing at school, I have a wide interest in music. But my first loves are the great Masses and Requiems. Those by Bach, Verdi and Mozart. Then comes Elgar's choral works and Vaughan Williams' *Sea Symphony* and lots of the symphonic repertoire. Some opera is important for me plus very early jazz and even Abba and Queen. So it was with great difficulty that I searched for a piece of music I could listen to with Mary. There was so much to choose from. I decided to begin with the *Dream of Gerontius* next session.

MB observations

15 June session

After my initial greeting enquiring how she was, Liz began to talk of the heartache and of feeling overwhelmed when she hears the Angel's aria. She feels as if she is being taken somewhere else. Held and gently supported – a difficult journey and then joy. We listened to it then together and I was aware of how Liz was feeling as the sound filled the room. When it was over I asked Liz what this piece meant for her in her life. She wondered if it had to do with her birth and the time immediately afterwards. Her birth had been a long labour and her mother had an 'illness' six weeks or so later and never seemed to recover. We are unclear what this was about. It might have been a bad attack of 'flu along with the onset of rheumatoid arthritis. She was told that her father had to come home from work during the day to tend to her mother and herself over the next months.

Liz's reflection on her first choice of music

Elgar's *Dream of Gerontius* is the story of a dying man's death and the journey with his guardian angel to Heaven. The angel sings about being loved and held right up to the moment of seeing God. The choir repeats part of the previous chorus 'Praise to the Holiest' and the harmony in the choir is breathtaking. The angel sings softly her farewells and then Gerontius moves on towards heaven with final repeated quiet Amens (so be it).

At the end of this work I feel the same as I do at the end of the *Messiah*. This is the culmination of three hours of another story – the Christian Faith. While I am listening and performing I can remove myself to 'another place'. I am away somewhere, away from my pain and my distress. Mary asked how I feel when I listen to such music. It is as though I am taken away from this place to a place where I feel weightless. It's a bit like lying in a swimming pool, just relaxed in the warm water with the sound wrapped all around me like a blanket. My breathing changes and becomes increased and shallower and my heart rate rises so that I begin to feel the pulse in my neck and right into my ears. If there is a change in rhythm and volume, especially if the music becomes more exciting, my skin begins to tingle and the sound if loud enough feels as if everything is blown out of my head (the pain of depression?) and I am completely somewhere else on a 'high' that I cannot explain. The problem of course is that I know that the piece will end and I will have to return to reality.

MB observations

8 July session

After welcoming Liz in the usual way as described above, we spent some time talking about the pain of being with her mother in the early years and perhaps her mother not being able to attend to her. (We were finding difficulty in arranging regular sessions at this point, which is an interesting parallel to Liz's mother not being available for her all those years ago.) Father was someone who held on to his feelings about music. He never sang in church she observed. Liz began to talk about how important choir was and is for her. We then agreed to work fortnightly after the holiday break, using music that Liz chose.

MB observations

4 August session

Liz arrived quite low and tearful. After greeting her, she talked a lot about how she might have been cared for in her early months. Grandma would have been there. She was a singer. (This is the first time that grandma has been talked about as someone around in her very early years.) When we talked about grandma she felt the pain of heartbreak in her chest and is going to bring in music that eases this.

MB observations

18 August session

When I saw Liz, I noticed that her face and body were a little more relaxed. After my initial welcome Liz announced that she had brought in music from the *Queen Symphony* by Tolga Kashif. We listened to this together and she noted that the ending had sorrow and joy in it together. We looked at what this might be about for her and how the ending was most significant for her. She reflected that when the conductor holds the audience it's as if 'time stops'. (This was felt in the room as she described it.) Liz then said that the sorrow is that time starts again. She described physical symptoms of wanting to cry as well as feelings of joy during the music – two feelings together. She left the recording of the *Queen Symphony* with me and may or may not bring a different piece of music.

It is interesting that the choice of music is now 'earthed' and more grounded, as it were, in the music of the *Queen Symphony* even though Liz talks of it as enabling her to escape into 'another world'. There may be a subconscious association with her grandmother here as Liz writes warmly of her reminding her of the old Queen Mary who was a real human being but who also belonged to 'another world' – a bygone world of order, manners and customs.

We then have the summer break. When we return there is the familiar restatement and deepening along with a further exploration of the dynamic constellation of the relationship between Liz, her grandmother and the feelings associated with her early years.

Liz's reflection on the *Queen Symphony* during the summer break

I first heard the *Queen Symphony* on the radio. I have always enjoyed Queen the pop group and years ago I thought Freddie Mercury was amazing. Perhaps this was because he was not afraid of being himself. I always had to be acceptable and the habit has stayed with me. Over the years I have tried to break out but now it feels a bit too late. This symphony is full of Queen popular tunes, orchestrated into a patchwork of harmony, glorious sounds woven into counterpoint which reaches a climax in the sixth movement. Orchestra and choir swell to the words 'Who wants to live forever?' Near the end there are two moments when a key change in the music twists the intensity so much that I feel this within my body to the extent that I begin to shudder. This music is rich in sound and emotion and seems to get right into the very core of me. Here again I can escape into my 'other world' and wallow in a blanket of sound which brings great comfort.

Return to therapy after the summer break

MB observations

9 September session

I welcomed her warmly and enquired how she was, having had the break. There was no music played at this session but we talked about her singing at Sunday School at the age of 8 or 9 and realising that her mother didn't recognise her talent, but the leader of the Sunday School did. She is going to do some writing and listen to more of the *Queen Symphony*.

MB observations

23 September session

Liz brought in the *Queen Symphony* again and we played some of it. There was talk about grandma caring for her and how her mother had not really seen her singing talent nor indeed her growing up.

Liz's writing, which I have not included in full, is a restatement of the context and feelings of the story of the Dream of Gerontius. It was as if she needed to restate and feel those feelings associated with this music before she could move on to the difficult and confusing stage which starts to open up new material.

Liz's reflection

4 October

The words are about being loved and held right up to the moment of seeing God. The choir repeats part of the previous chorus 'Praise to the Holiest in the Height'. The harmony from the choir is breathtaking. The angel softly sings her farewells and then Gerontius moves onwards towards Heaven. There are final repeated quiet 'Amens' until the last five bars where the 'Amen' is slowed down then gets loud to 'forte' and then a 'diminuendo' down to the end.

MB observations

8 October session

We did not listen to music today. Liz wanted to talk about the grief and anger around leaving her first marriage. There was a lot of pain and guilt around, which she hadn't mentioned before.

MB observations

20 October session

This was quite a confusing session. Liz arrived without the music CD she had wanted to play, the third movement of Beethoven's *Seventh Symphony*, the very wild and abandoned *Apotheosis of the Dance*, but she had selected by accident and played the first movement of Dvorak's *Second Symphony* instead. She then forgot to bring it!

I hummed the main tune from the first movement for her and she agreed that this might be the one. (It is interesting that I chose correctly. There could have been right-brain to right-brain resonance going on between us here, but this will be discussed more fully later.)

Liz was looking very lost and depressed and I enquired what music might be helpful for her. She replied that we might play the one I had la-lalled to her. She remembered then that she had listened to this passage from Dvorak's First Symphony with her mother. It had introduced the reading of *Nicholas Nickleby* as a serial on children's hour that she listened to with her. Liz had enjoyed it so much that her mother wrote to the BBC and found out what it was and bought the record for Liz who was then about nine years old.

This realisation brought a lot of confused feelings into the room for Liz. She realised how much her mother and father had really cared for her but she was also angry with them for 'not caring' enough for her in her earlier years. She was struggling with these conflicting feelings in the room. We talked of how these feelings she was struggling with were needing to be brought to words. Maybe we needed to work more with the music to bring these conflicting feelings to some sort of resolution. It is of note that some of the painful confused feelings in the room were not only to do with the realisation that her mother and father had bought this recording of Dvorak especially for her but that her grandmother had died just before her eleventh birthday. Being 11 years old was full of pain and confusion for Liz.

Liz's reflection on the Dvorak symphony

28 October

These minutes I spent with my mum listening to the Dvorak, while my dad and sister were at work, must have been a special time. When I look back, any time she had for me only was rare, so perhaps my present sadness is about not having enough 'special times' and wishing we could have had more.

Interestingly I have strong memories of how my parents' home felt and I now realise that in some aspects I try to re-create the same atmosphere in my own home. While I am planning new decoration I don't realise what I am doing until the work starts. We have recently had our sitting room decorated. I love dark rich colours and searched for weeks through many pattern books. Every book I looked at had light pale colours. But at last I found one – grey/purple with a hint of green background with the lines making a large diamond pattern in gold. I am having purple curtains that pick out a light purple shade from the newly covered suite that has flowers and leaves – lovely. It's not quite finished but even now I can tell it's just what I want cosy, warm and welcoming. I hate strong lights at home. Only the hall and the kitchen have bright lights. I like lamps in the sitting room and an adjustable light in the dining room that can be altered to whatever mood I'm in. A lot of this goes back to gas lights in my grandma's house. Gas lights give a different light, they are never still and move with the draft from an opening door. It makes different types of shadows but I don't remember ever being afraid. There is also a noise of the gas coming through the mantle. I just loved it.

MB observations

3 November session

Liz was much more lively this week. We talked of the confusion of the Dvorak/ Beethoven and how the musical mix-up was now resolved. (I noted that the Beethoven was a wild very energetic piece and the Dvorak movement was slow and reflective.) Through the confusion a middle place seemed to have been reached and something resolved. We listened to the Dvorak again and Liz told me that she has written of what it evoked in her and is recreating the atmosphere in the present in her home decorating using the colours she associated with the warm atmosphere in her parents' and grandparents' homes.

MB observations

17 November session

Liz arrived with writing about grandma and a very full description of what kind of person she was and what her relationships were with Liz's mother and grandfather. The following is an outline of some of the main features of this story.

Liz's reflection

13 November

My grandmother was born in 1883. I was nearly 11 when she died of bowel cancer and her funeral was on my 11th birthday. These are some of the memories of her during the first ten years of my life.

My grandmother was a good singer and when she was young she went round the local chapels singing short choral pieces. My mother was born in 1906 and my grandmother was pregnant before she married. This embarrassed my mum so much over the years that she always said that she was younger than her actual age. It also explains why she nagged me so much about the difficulties that could happen to young girls who get pregnant before they get married!

My grandfather was a demanding man and according to my mother he always got what he wanted. But I remember her standing up for herself and when I stayed with them if she did not like what he said, she would tell him. My mother always said that when grandma got the vote she had been known to vote the opposite to him just to spite him!

I remember my grandmother as grey haired but still very upright. She used to remind me of the old Queen Mary. We used to visit as a family on Sunday afternoons and stay for tea. In the summer there were always daisies to pick from the lawns and the 'rec' to explore. This was the park at the bottom of the back garden.

When I was 7 I went to stay for over a month with my grandma while my mum was in hospital and I have all sorts of memories of this time. It was summer and I went to school in the village. I think I liked it there. There were many happy memories of grandma doing my hair in plaits, my mum only did it in bunches. I remember playing in the sunshine on warm evenings and soapy baths and how she was able to put spiders out of the bedroom window. In the mornings I would wake up to the smell of frying tomatoes and bacon. Every time I cook these at home the aroma takes me back.

I remember when I was there I was not well and my grandma made elderflower tea. It tasted awful and it looked like bits of cauliflower floating and sitting in the bottom of the cup of warm tea. I don't remember being ill for long! It either worked or the thought of it made me feel better immediately.

I always enjoyed going to my grandma's. She cooked lovely dinners and made wonderful cakes. Sunday tea was always a treat. In the summer we always went for a walk after tea. Just up the road from where she lived were fields with flowers and butterflies and birds. Grandma always brought grandpa's walking stick so she could shoo away the cows. I always picked lots of wild flowers and gran would put them into little vases that stood on the dresser.

But after all this I had to return home. I can still picture gran standing at the gate watching us walk down the road. I would keep glancing back and at the corner we would wave goodbye. While I am typing this I can still feel that ache in my body – 'I don't want to go home . . . I don't want to go home'. I remember the dark winter nights watching the lamp posts going by and knowing that each one was taking me further away from my gran's house. The contrast was enormous, from peaceful village country living back to an inner city housing estate. Home meant strict rules: 'You can't do this', 'You can't go there', 'Be in on time', 'I don't like this friend of yours'. It was total control and I was desperate for some sort of freedom. I felt suffocated. I could not breathe. It must have been about this time around 8 or 9 when I began my other imaginary life! I was always sent to bed early so I would read or sing music from school. I began to imagine little friends coming to see me to talk to me. I don't remember now who they were or what they talked about but as long as the conversations lasted they were real to me.

My grandma was a very special person, someone I never really got to know. My regret is that I never spoke to her as an adult. I feel we would have had lots to talk about. My mum always said that my gran would have understood and supported me at the time of my divorce. All my life I have loved and remembered this woman as a strong part of my early years. I didn't realise until now just how important she was. I knew how to hide feelings and when she died just before my 11th birthday, no-one knew I was grieving. I told no-one, it got buried away.

MB observations

17 November session continued

After discussing much of this material with Liz I explained to her that what might be happening was that she was beginning to remember all this material because of us listening to music together. Within our relationship her right-brain material was being engaged with and these early good memories of grandma were now being processed and coming to words, perhaps for the first time.

I asked Liz what she understood about what might be happening through working with music. She replied that she is discovering pleasant memories. The loss is still there. What I thought about but didn't say at this point was that she has remembered taking leave of grandma and is beginning to grieve over her death but then recalls returning to mother who now has the stick for her arthritic illness.

There would have been much grief and rage about the death of grandma and the rage of going back to mother who was ill and still couldn't care for her as she longed to be cared for. The therapeutic task would be to hold the good feeling memory of grandma in conversation between us, which might begin to ameliorate the pain, guilt and loneliness of returning to her parents' home.

MB observations

30 November session

This started as a very uncomfortable session for Liz. She seemed confused and was finding everything a bit hard. This confusion and bewilderment was in the room. She then remembered sitting next to her mother on the bus. Her face lightened as she described the silky texture of her mother's dress and the diamond patterning of green, red and purple. She spoke of the warm cosy feeling of sitting next to her mother. Liz would have been about 5 or 6 at the time. I was aware of the warmth of this memory of being and feeling close to mother filling the room. I also recalled silently that she had decorated her living room in a purple diamond-patterned wallpaper which had felt warm and cosy!

MB observations

15 December session

Liz talked of being very busy leading up to Christmas. She then remembered Christmas with mum and the excitement on Christmas Day, sitting at the top of the stairs waiting to come down. She said she would do some more writing over the Christmas period before we next met on 5 January 2004.

Liz's reflection

29 December

I have seen Mary twice during December. The first time we talked about my mum and the pleasant memories I still hold. It is not the big event nor the dramatic moment that comes to mind but more the feel of being out with mum on a summer's afternoon or the close feeling of going shopping with her on the trolley bus. I remember warm days; she would sit close to me on the bus. I remember the feel of her dress; it was printed with squares in a diagrammatic design all in different colours of green, red and purple. All the squares were edged in black and pulled left and right so that the squares were nearly diamonds. It was made in very silky/crepe fabric which, even on hot days, felt very cool to the touch. The feel of her sitting close to me was wonderful. Just she and I . . . no distractions. I had her all to myself. This must have been a time of better health for her. I would have been about 5 or 6.

Another time when my mother showed understanding of my frame of mind was at Christmas. Christmas morning was a time of great excitement. She would let me get into her bed while my dad made the fire to warm the sitting room before I was allowed down to see my presents. I would sit at the top of the stairs and call over to my dad 'Has he been?' I was so excited I was almost unable to move. I would come down one step at a time giggling away until at last I would peep around the door. There would be the sight of parcels piled high on one of the easy chairs. Thinking of Christmas reminds me of what I am doing this Christmas.

At the beginning of December I sang the *Messiah* with the choral society. I am really mindful now of how I might feel during the performance. I was determined to sing every note and not get carried away by the effect of this music. We only had three rehearsals so I savoured every minute and looked forward to the concert night. The concert hall was three quarters full and the soloists were top professionals. I now sit in a space with room for a music stand to hold my score as I cannot hold my music and support myself with my walking stick. Somehow this seems to have freed up the physical action of my singing. Every chorus went like a dream. I enjoyed every note from the first chord of the Overture. Towards the end of 'Worthy is the Lamb that was Slain' there is a great build up of tension leading to the great 'Amen' at the end. By the time we reached the last page I was somewhere else. To be in the centre of all this glorious singing and the orchestra playing at full throttle takes me to this other *place.* At the pause, three bars from the end, the momentary silence just feels like the world has stopped for an instant. Everything has stopped – the music, the singing, the pain, the memories. I want to stay here yet I know I have to return to reality. We are coming to the end. Two bars from the end an '**Amen**': the final bar '**Amen. . . . . .**' Our conductor holds the final note waving his arm at us to sustain the volume of sound as long as we dare. I run out of breath and gasp for another while still holding this last sounding note. Before we finish I can see people smiling and clapping, standing up and cheering. The applause is deafening . . . It's wonderful . . . I struggle to hold back the tears and then we are breathing and laughing and smiling at each other. The sound of the applause rings in my ears. I stand there on the platform looking at the audience. I can see the smiling faces and hear the cheering and the whistling. The soloists come back on stage again, the orchestra stands up yet again and finally our conductor signals our final acknowledgement. It's over and I find myself back in the world that I struggle to live in. The battle continues. I will not give up! Music keeps me alive and helps me cope.

MB observations

5 January session

Liz arrived with much pain in her limbs. She moved very quickly to talk about her writing on her experience of the *Messiah*. She had also brought in photographs of her mother in the diamond-patterned dress she had described at the end of last year.

When she talked about the performance of the *Messiah* it was almost overwhelming for her. She could hardly speak. I encouraged her gently to try to do this, to try and regulate her breathing so that she had some sense of control in her body; a little affect regulation! She talked more about her mother and how excited she was as a child on Christmas morning. We then talked about the sadness of her mother's death when Liz was 30 and how her mother was just beginning to accept her as an adult. We talked with sorrow about the relationship with her mother that she would have missed.

MB observations

19 January session

Liz again arrived in some pain but the tone of her arrival was less depressive. She began by talking about an oil painting she was engaged in. It was a garden scene with buddleia and butterflies.

This artwork is running alongside the time it is taking to explore and understand better what her experience is in a given piece of music. Liz's experiential process seems to be slowly emerging from music alone through artwork towards words in the room with me. This multimedia therapeutic engagement will be discussed more fully in the next chapter.

Returning to the content of the session, we explored how there was no place for verbal expression of self-in-relationship when she was growing up. She said that she had felt that there was no self to express. The only self was her mother's when she was growing up – a kind of cloned self! We then listened to the first chorus of the *St Matthew Passion* together which she had brought in to the session.

Liz's reflection

1 February

I am not well at the moment. I have a virus infection in my throat, so I have had to cancel my session with Mary. I am listening to some music instead and I will write about it.

We have a big concert coming up and we will be performing Bach's *St Matthew Passion*. When I was last with Mary we listened to the Prologue into the first chorus. There is a strong pulse beat and I am aware of the flowing crotchet/quaver rhythm in the bass line. We have 16 bars introduction and then the chorus comes in. 'Come ye daughters, share my mourning'. This is so beautiful it makes my toes curl. The sound fills my body and head and for a few seconds blasts out all the stuff in there which seems to drag me down. There is a build up in the orchestra and then we get the tune. Such beautiful words and a lovely line to sing, which goes on until the end of the movement. The final chord completely enthrals me.

MB observations

16 February session

We talked of the Bach chorus and dying. I was silently recalling the deaths of Liz's mother and grandmother while I was reading her writing and her focus on 'Come ye daughters, share my mourning'. There was grief and sorrow in the room.

MB observations

23 February session

Liz came in feeling very low. She felt 'down in the dumps'; her legs and body were hurting. She felt that going to bed and sleeping was all she could do that would help. She brought some paintings – a seascape and the buddleia picture. She intends to do a course on drawing. She was brighter when she left.

Liz's reflection

24 March

I have been depressed for the last two weeks or more. When I saw Mary last time we talked about my childhood and how I might have felt as a small child. I decided that I should write something to remind me of what some of my pain might be about. It feels as if it might be about some of the loss, loneliness and emptiness all those years ago; the pain in my heart that I could not talk about, the pain that I now feel in my body. *My Returning Journey* is about this.

> *My Returning Journey*
>
> When I enter the tunnel, I must remember
> Who it is who is suffering.
> I am a babe in arms, with no arms to hold me
> I am alone in a lonely place
> No sound, no music, no voices
> My little body is in pain
> Breathing is difficult, pain in my chest
> Why do I feel like this? I have no words
> I want it to go away forever, but it still keeps coming back.
> Curtains are drawn, nothing to see, nothing but brick walls
> Cannot escape, just have to sit here and wait
> So very tired. Have to sleep. Might feel better when I wake
> Sleep takes me to a peaceful place
> I am a tiny child, I am unable to process what is happening to me
> Circumstances put me here, I blame no-one
> Whatever I feel as I grow up
> How I feel is not my fault.
> I see the tunnel behind me
> Again I emerge exhausted
> I must remember that all this was in the past
> And not happening now
> I look at my tiny child with compassion
> I hold her close and share my warmth
> I must always remember my tiny child is blameless
> I must hold, protect, and love this child with unconditional love.

To help me through this time I have been thinking about what I could listen to between my therapy sessions with Mary. I looked through my CD collection and had difficulty deciding which CD to choose. While I was out shopping I spotted a CD and bought it on impulse. It was the music from the third film of the *Lord of the Rings* trilogy, *The Return of the King*. I loved this film with all the story lines brought together. The piece of music which made the most impact upon me was *The White Tree.*

What I remember best was what was happening in my body. The movement starts quietly with strings playing. This makes me feel calm. The tempo then changes and I can feel my breathing changing. The pulse in the music becomes more insistent and I seem to be waiting for the repeated theme to come. Each time the main chord changes it moves the music on, driving it forward; building up to a tremendous crescendo. My breathing changes, my heart quickens, I cannot sit still. I want to conduct, count, physically feel the beat. There is then a dramatic moment when every instrument, the strings, the brass, get faster and faster, until the moment of climax, when all the instruments along with gongs and percussion stop. At this moment I feel release, like I have been set free to fly. The music carries on taking me along weightless in the air. Until the moment of 'whoosh' at the end. But then it's finished. I feel I have been taken to a special place, away from the world I know, leaving me breathless but knowing that the feelings from deep inside me are comforted by this glorious music. I don't think I quite know how to describe this ending.

When I saw Mary again we talked about listening and singing and what each meant for me. For me there is a difference between listening to music and taking part in a performance. Firstly, as a listener the main physical feeling is detachment. I am here and the music is over there. I am an observer and the music comes at me and then I respond. The initial feelings are nearly always the same. There is excitement so that my breathing changes and there is a sensation in my chest area of being locked up in a tense spasm bringing pain which seems to spread all over me. Sometimes I cry and I don't know what to do with myself so I have to wait until the moment passes.

When I am performing all the dynamics are different. First I am seated in the middle of a large choir with an orchestra just feet away. The sound is different because I am behind the orchestra. This actually alters the sound balance and sometimes we do not hear the soloists clearly due to the acoustics in the hall. This said, it never alters the impact of the performance. I am in the middle of a glorious sound community, when we all get going it's wonderful. I feel part of something amazing, voices blending in harmonies, with the orchestra playing away like mad making the whole thing *perfect.* So when it gets to a particularly lovely passage which I know will affect me I have to make sure I keep breathing correctly and keep counting the bars to ensure my singing voice does not disappear. My head becomes full of sound, the louder the sound the better. This seems to push out my depression and all I can hear is this glorious sound that I want to go on forever.

The physical act of singing, of producing the sound depends on good breathing. Deep breathing from the lower chest and then pushing out the sound with the singing voice is like expelling not just the words but the trapped, tightly held thoughts, feelings and also pain. The endings of some works are frequently difficult. While I sing I am in a different place, away from how I feel. But at the end I have to come back and face reality. For all my life I have escaped to music for respite. It has taken me to another world. When I perform I am not an observer listening from the outside, I am involved in all ways using my senses. My ears hear the sound of the music and I learn how to respond at the right time. My eyes watch the conductor to see the beat and learn when to come in and how to finish the words properly. My eyes also read the words and the notes that enable me to sing the notes with *my* voice. I feel much blessed to have this avenue to express my inner thoughts and who I really am.

MB observations

15 March session

Liz wrote a great poem *My Returning Journey* that she brought with her. We talked about this at some length. We then spoke about her writing on listening and singing and how she experiences these musical experiences differently. We then spoke at length about the music 'The White Tree'. This is about movement and becoming alive – like a bird flying, soaring.

MB observations

30 March session

Liz looked quite unwell. She is recovering from a virus. Her concert is on Sunday and she may not be able to sing, which distresses her greatly.

MB observations

25 April session

Liz arrived very bright and lively. We talked about how beautiful the trees were on her journey here and she remarked how beautiful the world was at the moment. She recalled that she had been listening to a very sparkling piece of music on the way to the session but had not heard the detail of what it was. She described it as a piano concerto with the pianist playing such joyful music with the notes seeming to collide and trip gleefully over one another in a torrent of happiness. What came into my head without having any knowledge of the radio programme that day was the Litolff *Piano Concerto*. I took the risk of singing the melody to her and she smiled broadly and confirmed that this was indeed the piece. We talked with some amazement and delight at this happy coincidence. How could I know this? Again this might be an example of right-brain communicating with right-brain! It is also interesting that her experience of listening or 'taking in' as nourishment has changed!

Happiness – the icing on the cake

Our work together came to an end on 22 June 2004. Liz felt she was in a better place than she had been when she first came. She was still in pain but there was a sense in which she had *it*, and *it* no longer had her. Liz wanted to write about where she thought she was now in her life and this chapter will end with this piece of writing. This will be followed by a reflection on the musical and therapeutic experience of this piece of work with Liz (*see* Chapter 11).

Liz's reflection on where I am today

3 July

In 1989 when I became ill with chronic fatigue I withdrew into an interior world and by 1991 I had entered therapy with my first therapist who held me in a wordless place with great care. I came to work with Mary in June 1995 until December 2002. Over these years I struggled with painful memories, depression and then fibromyalgia. Until recently I used music to withdraw into, using it as a big warm blanket. Over the past twelve months, with Mary's help, I now listen to music in a different way. I listen not only with my ears but by monitoring the sensations in my body. Music is now much more than a 'comfort blanket'. It gives me a way of focusing on the physical pleasure of the flowing sounds which feel really alive on those days when I am able to see the horizon, as it were, as well as being there for me when I am sad and depressed. A recent find is the Saint-Saëns *Organ Symphony*. If I am out in the car I like to turn up the volume and hear the full blasts of the sound so that it blows my ears out!! Another discovery is the Litolff *Piano Concerto No 2* (must be played by Peter Donaghue because of his sparkling performance). It makes me want to smile and I cannot sit still. I love the way the pianist slips the notes on the runs. It's so joyous I want it to go on forever. My last find is the film music by Howard Shore for *The Lord of the Rings*. I have always loved film music but I have found nothing to compare with this music from *The Lord of the Rings*. I find that my every mood is in this music somewhere and one of my favourite pieces is 'The White Tree', from the *Return of the King*. This CD is the story of good over evil, of journey in the full sense of the word. It could be a story of each person as they journey through life. Like Frodo on his journey we have battles, but ours are with our thoughts and fears, our feelings, pain and suffering and like Frodo the journey continues. Every day we fight a battle of some sort and we also can find help and support through partners, friends, relatives, faith, work, hobbies . . . not forgetting doctors and therapists!

When I am listening to music now I experience a full circle of feelings, a richer experience. Before this last year in therapy I would have left it at that and accepted that the feelings were *in the music*. Now I recognise that the feelings are not only in the music but are in *my own head and body*. This is very helpful information as I can now monitor what I listen to and protect myself from sounds and sights that I know from experience could cause trauma.

I feel I have travelled a long way in the last few years and my understanding of myself and why I have struggled so hard all my life is now at a level at which I am more able to deal with whatever the situation I find myself in. I have all this lovely music to help ease my depression and now also bring joy and light into my life. I will always keep music near me. It is the most important item in my life's haversack.

CHAPTER 11

Reflection on the two-part invention

Reflection and integration of ideas on the experience of listening to music in psychotherapy

In this chapter we will reflect upon the two-part invention from a therapeutic perspective. We will consider how Liz's early capacity for *communicative musicality*, or moving sympathetically with her first carers through sound and motion, was an important dynamic strand which was imprinted in her developing mind or brain. This strand is held to be central in her healing and integrative process.

After a lengthy period of therapeutic engagement for Liz from 1995–2002, our work together came to an end. However, Liz returned to therapy after a break of six months having been re-traumatised at a pain clinic. During the six-month break she had also been diagnosed with fibromyalgia. When she returned to therapy Liz first chose music, then painting and then words as media of communication.

Liz had first gone into therapy in the early nineties following the death of her father. It would seem that although she had made good progress during her first therapeutic encounter with my colleague and subsequently in therapy with me, there were many aspects of her early traumatic experience that had remained un-integrated. It could be that Liz was an example of someone who needed more than verbal psychotherapy in order to engage with her very early trauma.

I am reminded that Daniel Siegel holds the view that the framing of mental images within therapy in a safe holding containment may involve both verbal and non-verbal modes of engagement. The processes of these representations may facilitate integration across the brain hemispheres, and lead to increased psychological integration in general. He writes:

'These representations or mental images may be manifested in an array of modalities, from various forms of perception (sight, hearing) to words. . . . this suggests that the interpersonal sharing of the internal experience in words alone may not be the core curative feature within therapy'; . . . also 'The sense of safety and the emotional "holding environment" of a secure attachment within a therapeutic relationship . . . may be essential for these integrative processes to *finally* occur within the traumatised person's mind.'[1]

It seemed that Liz needed verbal psychotherapy and a safe holding environment for this multi-modal integration of early parts of her attachment experience to begin to become operative and be worked with.

In writing about this early attachment period and how our infant brains receive and encode relational information about the world around us, and the carers close to us, Turnbull and Solms write that:

> 'The goal-directed, rational, realistic, selective and chronologically sequenced way of remembering, that we rely upon as adults is thus not characteristic of those early years of life. . . . Since the goal-directed frontal system plays an important part in *controlling* encoding and consolidating processes too, it seems highly likely that the memory traces of young children are actually *stored* differently from the way they are stored in adult brains. If something is encoded in one form, it is more difficult to retrieve it accurately in another form.'[2]

This would account perhaps for the difficulty in reaching this early multi-modal relational state of being-in-relationship during her first period of psychotherapy. Perhaps she needed to be met in a more focused way through *enhanced communicative musicality*, that is, music added to the innate ability, which functions from birth, for being able to move sympathetically with another.[3] Her psychotherapy needed another kind of coding, perhaps the sound of music, to reach this particular mental trace of being-in-relationship with a carer who was important for her well-being and emotional development.

It is interesting to note that when Liz and I first met in 1995 we did try to communicate through shared playing in the pentatonic scale. (One form of the pentatonic scale is found by playing only on the black notes of the piano.) This was because Liz was finding it very difficult to communicate verbally, except for a very few words. This playing in the pentatonic scale was hard for Liz but she stayed with it and found that a lot of grief and sorrow seemed to have been met. If this grief and sorrow was indeed encoded in musical sounds and phrases this might have been a significant episode of relating with me which resonated with the very early experience with her mother who later became ill. This joint improvisation or active music therapy has been referred to earlier in this book.

Liz could not of course remember in words what had happened to her after she was born, when her mother was no longer there for her emotionally but living under the same roof. This loss, however, would have been felt and imprinted in her developing brain. She had begun to 'know' mother in this close sensing way from the beginning of her life in the womb, but this feeling and sensing knowledge had now become confused, perhaps by being handled by an array of different carers, including Grandma of course. It must be noted that Liz's mother was still quite frail at this time and needed much help and support from father and other carers.

These sensations of loss were imprinted in her developing right brain and the accompanying sorrow and bewilderment felt at the first loss of her mother and then grandmother after six weeks or so would have been encoded there in implicit memory. Wilkinson writes:

> 'Implicit memory is the source of the deeply founded ways of being and behaving that govern an individual life. These hidden depths are the early established patterns, recorded in the implicit memory store of the early developing right hemisphere.'[4]

As a small infant, Liz would perhaps have felt quite lost, confused and traumatised. People came and went and continuity was re-started only for it to disappear. We now know that the first months of life are vitally important for how our brains develop and how we relate to others in the world. Green, Wilkinson, Gerhardt, Solomon and Siegel, Cozolino, Corrigall and Wilkinson, and Schore are just a few authors who have considered and studied the effects of such early damage of people who enter into psychotherapy.[5–11]

Schore writes:

> 'The essential task of the first year of a human's life is the creation of a secure attachment bond between the infant and the primary caregiver.'[12]

He writes that after the infant's developmental milestone at about two months, with the maturation of the occipital cortex, there is a dramatic progression of the infant's social and emotional capacities. This is when the mother's face and reflecting gaze become especially important for the baby. This would be around the time of early confusion for Liz. Although Schore is writing here primarily about the visual mode of engagement between mother and child, this reflexive engagement 'affect synchrony' applies to sound also.[13] He continues:

> 'In this process of "affect synchrony" . . . the intuitive mother initially attunes and resonates with the infant's resting state, but as this state is dynamically activated (or de-activated or hyper-activated) she fine tunes and corrects the intensity and duration of her affective stimulation in order to maintain the child's positive affective state. The primary caregiver thus facilitates the infant's information processing by adjusting the mode, amount, variability and timing of stimulation to its actual temperament. These mutually attuned *synchronized* interactions are fundamental to the ongoing affective development of the infant mental physiological abilities.'[12]

Liz had a bewildering first year of life. She could not process these early losses because, although all the brain structures are in place and ready to be developed, the brain is not mature enough at that early period of infancy to process these experiences into thought.

But there would have been early experiences perhaps of mother, grandmother and carers engaging in baby songs with her which had a narrative dynamic motion of a beginning, a middle and an end. There would have been early right brain memory traces of patterns of *communicative musicality*, that is of moving sympathetically with another but the continuity of this dynamic process was fragile. She had also learned through her brain/body that this human dynamic of *communicative musicality*; these moving sounding patterns with a significant other could disappear at any time. Life was confusing and uncertain for Liz at the very early time when these important brain processes were coming on stream as it were.

Later in childhood this early but fragile musical patterning of beginning, middle and end was further established through her singing in the school choir. Here she would find that her confused feelings of love and loss could be ordered and experienced **in music** in a way that was meaningful and which made sense to her. These feelings could now be thought about. She also learned that she had a measure of control over this dynamic of love and loss and that she could choose to experience her feelings through this narrative of beginning, middle and end in singing or listening to music.

Liz had had no such control over this dynamic narrative of love and loss as a baby. As she grew older, along with enjoying and learning more about music Liz used passages of music as source templates for this dynamic processing of love and loss. She was safe in music and her adult experience of music had been built upon the *communicative musicality* she experienced through the intermittent dynamic loving interactions with her mother and grandmother.

In the last chapter, Liz finished her writing with 'Where I am today'. Here she describes how before the last year of therapy she accepted that the feelings were *'in the music'* but now she recognises that not only are they in the music they are in *'my own head and body'*.

In *Coming Into Mind* Wilkinson writes that traumatic experiences, either in infancy or later can sometimes be so overwhelming that they are put out of mind. They are dissociated. Of early traumatic experience she writes:

> 'Traumatic experience becomes encoded in implicit memory, unavailable to the conscious mind.'[14]

When Liz writes that the feelings she experienced were *'in the music'* she is describing a state of dissociation. Music was the place where not only did she find patterning which held the dynamic process of love and loss noted above, she had unconsciously put her warm loving tender feelings, particularly those associated with love and loss, there also. These warm good feelings were the intense, loving, tender feelings that she found overwhelming and unable to cope with because they were linked with sorrow and early separation from her mother, father and grandmother. But what of the pain and sorrow she had experienced as an infant?

What was obvious was that Liz as an adult in the consulting room was in considerable pain due to fibromyalgia and this too would have had an emotional component in her brain or mind. What we now know is that early traces of mental pain and loss are stored in implicit memory but may be felt over the years in the body. Scaer, quoted in Wilkinson's *Coming Into Mind*, lists bodily symptoms suffered by those who have experienced traumatic stress.[15] Among the illnesses listed are neuromuscular symptoms, fibromyalgia and chronic fatigue syndrome (ME).

How might fibromyalgia and chronic fatigue syndrome be linked to early traumatic stress?

It is suggested here that the early unconscious traces in Liz's brain or mind, the sensations and feelings of loving and painful loss, were gradually dissociated into music, and Liz's body. As she grew older the dissociation could no longer be fully contained in the mind and it divided itself between mind and body.

Although Liz felt warm good feelings in her body while singing and listening to music paradoxically Liz's body held the pain of fibromyalgia when she was not caught up in performing or listening to music. Solomon, writing on the body as a container of early traumatic memories, states:

> 'The psyche is . . . unable to process it and is liable to store trauma in the body memory. . . .The patient's body has had to share the burden of the traumatising experience with the psyche. It is as if the psyche could not tolerate the full impact, or else could not make sense of the experience except by rendering it into organic form, or because the traumatising history had such real toxic effects on the physical system.'[16]

It is as if the psyche, in patients like Liz, separates the good and bad feelings. The good feelings are held in music and the bad in the body. Jung described these dissociated aspects of the personality as 'autonomous splinter psyches', which became split off because of traumatic experience.[17]

But how were we to begin to undo this trauma of early losses which brought about this dissociation into music and the body, where the intensity associated with good feelings was held in music and the pain of the bad feelings was felt in Liz's body? Wilkinson writes:

> 'Trauma needs to be undone in the brain. Although the self is fundamentally associative and relational, dissociative defences may come into play to protect a patient from overwhelming affect at a time when it would be truly unbearable. Their affects lie symbolically between "in mind" and "out of mind"'.[18]

The task would be to allow these dissociated early sensations and feelings, these traces in implicit memory and held in music and the body, to be experienced together in the room in as safe a way as Liz could manage without being re-traumatized. This would mean *following* Liz's choice of music and *tracking* carefully the movement of the feelings and sensations that Liz communicated to me within the therapeutic process. It would also mean making appropriate interpretations but being led by Liz on every occasion. This would allow Liz to bring the feelings and associations with music and the body to mind as explicitly as Liz could manage. There are, of course, issues concerning therapeutic technique involved here in order to avoid re-traumatization and we will consider these in Chapter 12.

For Liz, in the past, the difficult feelings and sensations she had had in relation to her early attachment figures and experienced as too overwhelming to be thought and talked about interpersonally needed to be placed in passages of music between 'in mind' and 'out of mind', where they could be experienced and tolerated but not worked with nor thought about. These early feelings and sensations were stored in implicit or unconscious memory. However, Liz's feelings of pain and weakness experienced throughout her adult life as ME and fibromyalgia, could have had their roots in her early feelings and sensations of pain and sorrow. They were 'in mind' in the sense that she was conscious of the pain every day but they were 'out of mind' because they were dissociated from their early roots. Referring to the encoding of early memories and their emergence in later life, Wilkinson writes:

> 'Traumatic experience affects both the encoding and recall of the memories associated with it. The earlier in life and the more sustained the traumatic experience is, the more likely this is to happen. Such traumatic experience becomes encoded in implicit memory, unavailable to the conscious mind. The body may hold the memory for the patient for many years until mind and psyche are strong enough to deal with the unbearable experience.'[14]

Music in the consulting room

We will now turn to music in the consulting room. Liz and I both experienced intense feelings in the music that she brought into the sessions. Before this last period of therapy, Liz seemed to use some music as a dissociative defence, as described above. This would mean that when Liz experienced feelings of containment and bittersweet longing in relation to particular pieces of music she was perhaps using music unconsciously as a medium to keep these feelings 'in mind' and also 'out of mind'. These feelings were 'in mind' because she temporarily experienced their intensity, but they were also 'out of mind' because they were dissociated from early real experience and stored in early implicit memory unavailable to words.

Liz's *later* memories which may have had their roots in the early traumatic experience of love and loss were successfully kept at bay, because in music they were never brought into mind by talking about these feelings and what they meant for her.

As therapy progressed these experiences moved from this kind of 'no man's land' in music and the body memory to explicit memory, that is, they were now linked with left hemisphere pathways and processes in the brain. Here they could be talked about and their meaning better understood for her. She was also able to talk more specifically about the joy, sorrow, pain and loss she had felt in relation to her mother and grandmother.

The other artistic media, her painting and poetry, were important symbols and markers of her journey into mind. The artwork and poetry that Liz engaged in only seemed to emerge after the experience of listening to music was well underway. Experiencing music in the consulting room could be seen as a developmental parallel mirroring the sequence of the development of the neuro-sensory systems, in that hearing is the first to be developed in the womb followed by vision;[19] words come on stream between one and two years after birth.

The conversation in any therapeutic session has a beginning, a middle and an end which is like the flow of a piece of music. But there was also something more going on. Returning to Trevarthen and Malloch's thinking,[20] there were lengths of time in any session when through the particular empathic engagement of mirroring gestures, shared glances and tone of voice 'communicative musicality' was at play. That is, there was a heightened empathy between us at these times and it is suggested here that this is when *transference* and *counter-transference* took centre stage. We will now consider the phenomena of *transference* and *counter-transference* more fully in this context of music within psychotherapy.

Transference, counter-transference and communicative musicality

Transference is the particular dynamic shapes of feeling and sensation felt by the patient. These feelings and sensations have been experienced in the patient's past in earlier relationships and are now 'put on' to or transferred on to the therapist. The therapist is then experienced by the patient as if they are that earlier person in certain aspects. That is, the patient then behaves and relates to the therapist as if they are the patient's mother, or father, or grandmother or some wonderful or fearsome figure from the past. In terms of communicative musicality, the patient responds to the musicality of the tone of voice and movement of the therapist as if they are the mother, or father or grandmother in the consulting room.

The main features of the process of transference are as follows:

- The patient's past experiences and feelings are redirected to the therapist.
- The patient then experiences the therapist as that figure from the past in certain aspects.
- The patient responds to the tone of voice and/or movement or expression of the therapist as if they *are* that person from the past.

The counter-transference describes the therapist's feelings in the consulting room when they meet the early feelings and sensation configurations that belong to the patient's earlier life. The first task for the therapist is to separate out which feelings belong to the therapist and which belong to the patient's transference. The therapist and the transferential figure, for example the patient's mother, or father or grandmother, etc. may share the particular tone of voice or shape and intensity of feeling and this needs to be worked with in the therapist's supervision and a measure of clarity achieved so that the therapeutic work can proceed. This means that the therapist must put their feelings about the transference to one side and respond to the communicative musicality of the patient. For example, if the patient is behaving towards the therapist as if they are an 'angel', the therapist must focus on the *need* of the patient for the therapist to hold this configuration. The patient may be feeling lost and helpless and it is this point of pain which must be borne by the therapist. The therapist may feel kind and beneficent but with a bit of self-reflection will soon realise that they are no angel!

The main features of the process of counter-transference are:

- The therapist monitors their own feelings being aware that the therapist's unresolved unconscious material will be in the music.
- A particular strand of feeling may be that which is transferred from the patient.
- This strong feeling may be added to the same kind of feeling that belongs to the therapist.
- The therapist holds both these feelings without reacting until they have separated out which aspects belong to him or herself and which aspects belong to figures from the patient's past.
- The process is clarified in supervision if necessary.
- The on-going communicative musicality of the therapy is the responsibility of the therapist whose task it is to hold the flow of strong feelings with as little disruption as possible.

In this 'playground' or 'habitus' for the transference and counter-transference in psychotherapy with Liz we sometimes listened to music together. When music came into the room in this way it could be called *enhanced* communicative musicality, that is, the actual practice of listening to passages of music within therapy. It must be emphasised that the music was brought into the sessions by Liz and will be discussed more fully in the next chapter.

Through listening to music in this context of *enhanced communicative musicality*, Liz's dissociative feelings were slowly undone in some measure in her brain. Siegel writes on representations of patients such as Liz who have suffered early trauma that:

> 'These representations or mental images may be manifested in an array of modalities, divided at the most basic level between the non-verbal and the verbal. The sense of safety and the emotional "holding environment" of a secure attachment within a therapeutic relationship . . . may be essential for these integrative processes to (finally) occur within the traumatized person's mind.'[21]

We will now consider Liz's early emotional development and what some of her experiences of communicative musicality might have been with her mother and grandmother.

Liz's early life

Before and after her birth Liz would have been drawn to the musical sound of her mother's voice as she perhaps sang to her and lulled her to sleep. Having got used to her mother's voice and how she was lovingly cared for both within and outside the womb in the first weeks, Liz 's mother was then absent for periods of weeks and months. Liz would have been confused and bewildered at this loss of the warm intimacy of her mother's voice and her touch.

As has been written above, these aural and tactile experience are stored in memory traces in the developing brain. Research has shown that the hearing capacity of the human foetus is fully developed at the age of four months and can hear the full range of his of her mother's voice.[22,23] However, not only is the foetus capable of hearing and listening to the mother's voice, and the physical sounds of her body,[24] but her voice, her body sounds and heartbeat leave traces in the infant's memory. Maiello writes:

> 'Not only are sounds perceived and listened to by the fetus but research has shown that both the rhythmical sounds produced by the mother's organism and her voice leave traces in her (his) memory.'

She also writes that her hypothesis is that:

> 'proto-forms of an experience of relatedness may develop between the fetus and his mother not only at the tactile, but also at the auditory level'.[25]

Maiello continues:

> 'The specificity of the voice with its personal inflections and modulations of each individual mother puts the fetus in touch not only with the uniqueness of her personality, but also with the general state of her mind as well as the fluctuations of her emotions . . . It is probable that he receives clues about her emotional states not only through biochemical fluctuations in her organism, but also at the vocal level.'[26]

Liz was born in her grandmother's house and would have had an early form of attachment to her in the weeks that she stayed there. When she left she 'lost ' her sense of continuity with this loving figure when she moved back home with her mother. But Liz was loved by her mother and father and well cared for, and seemed to settle, as far as is known. It is to be noted that she would perhaps have known her grandmother's singing voice from this early time as grandmother sang a lot. But the loss of grandmother's constant presence, and her return to mother in her own home who became increasingly ill and fragile, was perhaps a traumatic loss which Liz would have found too difficult to process in her infant brain.

Wilkinson writes that 'early brain development is adversely affected by dissociative experience in the earliest relationships'[27] and quotes substantial research to underpin this statement. Teicher has found that there are impaired connections between the right and left hemispheres of the brain in the corpus callosum which connects the two hemispheres of the brain.[28] But Schore is quoted as holding the view that 'dissociation is best understood as a loss of connectivity within the right hemisphere'.[29] This hemisphere is involved in processing sound and feeling within the body.

From both these perspectives, it means that how the brain organises and internalises relationships and events in the outside world is affected by losses which the infant brain/psyche cannot understand or process. The infant brain/psyche in these circumstances adapts in the only way it can by shutting down what is confusing and overwhelming. What was confusing and overwhelming for Liz was her relationship with her mother and then her grandmother.

Liz's childhood

As she grew through childhood Liz seemed deeply attached to her grandmother with her elderflower tea and lovely cakes. She spent over a month with her when she was seven. However, she belonged to her father and her mother. Her mother was in physical pain and enveloped in sadness a lot of the time and Liz hated returning to this atmosphere in later childhood. She really loved the visits to her grandmother who sang and loved wild flowers. This was a confused state of being-in-relationship and during this time she had imaginary friends in whom she confided. (Who else could she trust?) This continued until Liz was nearly 11. Then her grandmother died and was buried on her birthday.

From this time of early adolescence her grief and sorrow became ever more etched in her brain. What could she do with all these confused deep feelings of love and sorrow? It would seem that the good experience of grandmother that had been felt in association with her and music became more dissociated because of grief after her death.

Perhaps Liz adapted to the loss of her grandmother by experiencing her presence, her loving way of being with her, through music. The sadness and feelings of lost loneliness were now increased in relation to her mother. In a sense they also belonged to her mother too in her continuing ill health. These losses and the grief that went with them became built into Liz's way of being in the world.

Writing on an 'Overview of the affective psychology of a secure attachment in healing trauma', Schore writes:

> 'The essential task of the first year of human life is the creation of a secure attachment bond of emotional communication between the infant and the primal caregiver. Within episodes of affect synchrony, parents engage in intuitive, non-conscious, facial, vocal, and gestural preverbal communications . . . In order to do this the mother must be psycho-biologically attuned to the dynamic crescendos and decrescendos of the infant's bodily-based internal states of arousal.'[30]

It is clear from the above description of Liz's early life that her early secure attachment bond of emotional communication was compromised by loss at a very vulnerable time when she could not process the loss of her grandmother's presence and the emotional attachment communication with her mother. Another vulnerable time in her emotional development was when she was 11 when her grandmother died and the dissociation process was continued.

The task therefore in therapy was to strengthen and rebuild an emotional scaffolding through interactive communicative experiences between us which allowed Liz to be more fully present in the world and not hidden in music or in her overwhelming physical pain. But how was this to be accomplished?

In *Coming Into Mind* Wilkinson writes that:

> 'The plasticity of the brain is a central concept underpinning the under-standings of both the development of the mind and the nature of the thera-peutic cure.'[31]

This means that although Liz is a mature woman in her 50s there is no reason why she should not benefit from therapeutic work relating to her early relation-ships. In support of this statement Wilkinson quotes Schore:

> 'The prefrontal limbic cortex retains the plastic capacities of early develop-ment throughout the lifespan thus making possible therapeutic change.'[32]

However, working in this inter-subjective way means that the therapist changes too. Wilkinson writes that working in a totally interactive experiential way in therapy affects both the brain/mind of the patient and therapist.

> 'This process of cure is not only the making of unconscious conscious as with interpretation but also the total interactive experience within both members of the analytic dyad. Through experience within the dyad, new entities are added to pre-existing connections in both brain-minds. Past is revisited at the level of the implicit, changing deeply founded ways of being and behaving then linked with present by means of transformative interpretation within the context of actual relational experience, leading to change in the nature of attachment. This way of working is at the heart of the response of the psychodynamic therapies to the insights that are emerging from affective neuroscience.'[31]

This writing has informed the practice of listening to music within psycho-therapy. Liz's aural, visual and verbal capacities which had been developing in infancy were fully engaged in the now mature adult through enhanced com-municative musicality. This practice in which Liz chose passages of music which we listened to together could have connected with traces of her early capacity for movement and empathic feelings. Trevarthen has named this capacity the Intrinsic Motive Pulse (IMP).[20] These traces would have been first built into her brain through communicative musicality with her mother and then her grandmother. However, as we grow through childhood, verbal language begins to come to the fore and we begin to express how we feel in words. Gestures and non-verbal modes of communication give way to spoken language. Trainer and Schmidt write:

'An emotional bond and the communication of positive and prohibitionary emotional information is essential for survival. Perhaps music evolved in order to further communication between infants and caregivers. As children develop other means of communication such as language, and as they learn to keep overt expressions of emotion under control, music may go "underground".'[33]

In this passage no distinction is made between music and communicative musicality. But as has been written above communicative musicality is with us throughout life and we are the richer for it. Music itself could be said to arise from the linking of musical sounds to human persons, first experienced as communicative musicality with our first carers. When we experience this linking as a sonorous narrative, with a beginning, a middle and an end, we experience music. When a further stage of intellectual/emotional complexity is then added to this developed form of communicative musicality we might be describing the *discipline* of music as we engage in informed listening, singing in a choir or playing a musical instrument.

Keeping in mind that this theoretical chapter is only part of a case study, we will now explore how the discipline of music made a difference in the course of Liz's therapy. In other words, we will consider in more detail the process of enhanced communicative musicality for Liz.

References

1 Siegel DJ (2003) An interpersonal neurobiology of psychotherapy: The developing mind and the resolution of trauma. In: MF Solomon and DJ Siegel (eds) *Healing Trauma*. WW Norton & Co., New York and London, p. 29.

2 Turnbull O and Solms M (2003) Memory, amnesia and intuition: A neuro-psycho-analytic perspective. In: V Green (ed.) *Emotional Development in Psychoanalysis, Attachment Theory and Neuroscience*. Brunner-Routledge, Hove and New York, p. 78.

3 Trevarthen C and Malloch S (2002) Musicality and music before three: Human vitality and invention shared with pride. *Journal of Zero to Three: National Center for Infants, Toddlers and Families*. **23** (1): 11.

4 Wilkinson M (2006) *Coming Into Mind*. Routledge, London and New York, p. 57.

5 Green V (ed.) (2003) *Emotional Development in Psychoanalysis, Attachment Theory and Neuroscience*. Brunner-Routledge, Hove and New York.

6 Wilkinson M (2006) *Coming Into Mind*. Routledge, London and New York.

7 Gerhardt S (2004) *Why Love Matters*. Brunner-Routledge, Hove and New York.

8 Solomon MF and Siegel DJ (eds) (2003) *Healing Trauma*. WW Norton & Co., New York and London.

9 Cozolino L (2002) *The Neuroscience of Psychotherapy*. WW Norton & Co., New York and London.

10 Corrigall J and Wilkinson H (2003) *Revolutionary Connections*. Karnac Books Ltd., London and New York.

11 Schore A (2003) *Affect Regulation and the Repair of Self*. WW Norton & Co., New York and London.

12 Schore A (2003) The Seventh Annual John Bowlby Memorial Lecture. In: J Corrigall and H Wilkinson (eds) *Revolutionary Connections*. Karnac Books Ltd., London and New York, pp. 13–14.

13 Papousek M and Papousek H (1995) Intuitive parenting. In: MH Bornstein (ed.) *Handbook of Parenting, Vol. 2: Ecology and Biology of Parenting*. Erlbaum, Hillsdale, NJ.

14 Wilkinson M (2006) *Coming Into Mind*. Routledge, London and New York, p. 61.

15 Scaer RC (2001) *The Body Bears the Burden: Trauma dissociation and disease*. Haworth Press, New York, London and Oxford. Quoted in: M Wilkinson (2006) *Coming Into Mind*. Routledge, London and New York, pp. 97–98.

16 Solomon H (2004) Self creation and the 'as if' personality. *Journal of Analytical Psychology*. **40**(5): 635–56.

17 Wilkinson M (2006) *Coming Into Mind*. Routledge, London and New York, p. 159.

18 Ibid, p. 94.

19 Lickliter R (2000) Atypical perinatal sensory stimulation and early perceptual development: insights from developmental psychobiology. *Journal of Perinatology*. **20**: 45–54.

20 Trevarthen C and Malloch S (2002) Musicality and music before three: human vitality and invention shared with pride. *Journal of Zero to Three: National Center for Infants, Toddlers and Families*. **23**(1): 16.

21 Solomon MF and Siegel DJ (2003) *Healing Trauma*. WW Norton & Co., New York and London, p. 29.

22 Tomatis AA (1981) *La Nuit Uterine*. Stock, Paris.

23 Prechtil HFR (1989) Fetal behaviour. In: A Hill and J Volpe (eds) *Fetal Neurology*. Raven Press, New York.

24 Macfarlane A (1977) *The Psychology of Childbirth*. Open Books Publishing Ltd., London.

25 Maiello S (2004) On the meaning of prenatal auditory perception and memory for the development of the mind: A psychoanalytic perspective. In: M Nocker-Ribaupierre (ed.) *Music Therapy for Premature and Newborn Infants*. Barcelona Publishers, Gilsum NH, p. 52.

26 Ibid, p. 53.

27 Wilkinson M (2006) *Coming Into Mind*. Routledge, London and New York, p. 9.

28 Teicher M (2000) Wounds that time won't heal: The neurobiology of child abuse. *Cerebrum*. **2** (4): 50–67. Quoted in M Wilkinson (2006) *Coming Into Mind*. Routledge, London and New York, p. 9.

29 Schore A (2005) Early relational trauma, disorganised attachment, and the development of a pre-disposition to violence. In: MF Solomon and DJ Siegel (eds) *Healing Trauma*. WW Norton and Co., New York and London, p. 113.

30 Schore A (2001) The right brain as the neurobiological substratum of Freud's dynamic unconscious: In: D Scharff (ed.) *The Psychoanalytic Century: Freud's legacy for the future*. Other Press, New York, p. 73. Quoted in M Wilkinson (2006) *Coming Into Mind*. Routledge, London and New York, p. 11.

31 Wilkinson M (2006) *Coming Into Mind*. Routledge, London and New York, p. 10.

32 Ibid, p. 11.

33 Trainer LJ and Schmidt LA (2003) Frontal EEG responses. In: I Peretz and M Zatorre (eds) *The Cognitive Neuroscience of Music*. Oxford University Press, Oxford, p. 321.

CHAPTER 12

Musical analysis of Liz's experience

Analysis of the musical and therapeutic processes

Enhanced communicative musicality

This chapter is an analysis of Liz's choices of music listened to in her psychotherapy sessions. The centrality of communicative musicality will be seen in the use of Malloch's categories of pulse, quality and narrative in the therapeutic engagement. These categories were originally used by Malloch to describe and identify more precisely what was going on in the relational communication through sound, gesture and movement between infants and mothers.[1] This work is based on Colwyn Trevarthen's research over many years into the psychobiology of infant–mother communication. In this chapter these categories will be used to identify more precisely what might have been going on in the music listened to by Liz and I in the consulting room.

Communicative musicality is also said to be present in the interpersonal psychotherapeutic engagement when the therapist's and patient's relationship seems to flow together and attune. It is suggested here that *enhanced* communicative musicality occurred when Liz and I listened together to the passages of music chosen by Liz. This listening to music seemed to heighten and support the dynamic relational flow between us.

Because communicative musicality is with us throughout life and not only in infant–mother communication, I will apply Malloch's categories of pulse, quality and narrative to the passages of music Liz chose to bring into the consulting room and to the musicality of the therapeutic engagement itself. The dynamic musical categories of pulse, quality and narrative of persons and music will be seen to overlap in this analysis.

Liz's first choice of music was the Angel aria from the *Dream of Gerontius* by Edward Elgar.

The Angel aria from the *Dream of Gerontius* by Edward Elgar

This is a narrative poem by John Henry Newman and set to music as an oratorio by Edward Elgar. It is about the dying of Gerontius and the journey of his soul to meet God. On this journey the soul is accompanied by an 'Angel' who has a female singing voice. It could be said that the angel's voice is being used symbolically as a bridge from one state of being to another state of being. Gerontius is a living human being nearing the point of death in the poem. His journey to meet God is about the transition from being human to being supernatural.

It is of interest here that Monika Nocker-Ribaupierre,[2] a music therapist who specialises in auditory stimulation after premature birth, writes of our first experience of the female voice as a bridge from our intra-uterine experience in the womb to our being born into the experience of the world outside the womb. Although this human journey is real and not symbolic, by describing the female voice of the mother as a *bridge*, she is using a metaphor which has a reality about it. The reality is that the infant hears the tone, timbre, rhythm and pitch of mother's voice from within the womb and then hears these same auditory features outside the womb when he or she is born. The auditory bridge is indeed real. It is the sound bridge *of* and *to* mother.

Nocker-Ribaupierre writes that this bridge from the auditory intra-uterine experience of the foetus to being an infant in the outside world is understood on several levels for both mother and infant. She describes how the foetus experiences *in utero*, the visceral sounds and the mother's heartbeat. She notes that the mother's heartbeat is a starting point for the relationship between rhythm and the human and its rhythm protects the newborn baby psychologically. She writes:

> 'This rhythm of the mother's heart beat protects the baby because it symbolizes security and reliable return ... The mother's voice is the basis for a more distinct impact in the relationship between the mother and the fetus. It is created not so much by the discursive but the presentative content of the voice and its emotional message is decisive. Sound, melody and the rhythm of the voice have an essential and formative psychological impact.'[3]

Nocker-Ribaupierre then lists how the mother's voice creates a bridge at several levels:

1 For the infant from the intra-uterine life to the extra-uterine life.
2 For the infant from the intra-uterine life through the technical life in the NICU to life at home.
3 For the mother from the experience of being pregnant to suddenly not being pregnant anymore.
4 For the emotional connection, the bonding process of both.[4]

Liz's choice of the Angel aria could be understood as symbolic of this early bridge from one state of being to another.

In the transference and counter-transference I could have represented the Angel alongside Liz, accompanying her on her journey into the unknown in the embodied world of where we are now. This might have been so because I could have been carrying the dynamic configuration of her mother and grandmother. These relational dynamics were present in the earlier therapeutic work done before Liz's visit to the pain clinic. The Angel could have become a symbol of her mother and grandmother.

It is of importance, though, that Trevarthen writes that it is not so much the content of the symbol but the ways in which the symbol is expressed that are important when considering an autobiography. Exploring *Who writes the autobiography of an infant?*, he states that he is less concerned with the symbolised contents of a life story and more concerned with the relational processes involved. He writes:

> 'The ways an infant seeks for experience, expresses interest and satisfaction or fear and confusion with what eventuates and above all the ways the child makes apparent to others the emotions of experience and evaluates from others' behaviour their sympathy and co-operation, all this might help explain what the human self and its memory comes from.'[5]

His thinking on the processes involved in any symbolisation would mean that, rather than putting emphasis on the content of the symbol in listening to music within psychotherapy, the ways of listening and seeing for Liz and myself would enable or disable her narrative of who was in the past and in the present in our relationship.

These ways of listening, the feelings and nuances of affect in the therapeutic transference and counter-transference, could be said to have been *enhanced* by the flow of music for both of us as we listened actively to the beautiful aria of the Angel. This serene vocal sound with its flowing comforting soothing shapes could have been reverberating with the early traces of the sonorous tones of her mother and then grandmother as a small child. These traces or nuances of sound would have been stored in implicit memory in Liz's right brain/mind.

Analysis of the shared listening experience

In terms of Malloch's categories of communicative musicality,[1] the pulse of the music was *slow and steady*, the quality *calm and serene* and the story or narrative that of a *transition from one state of being in the world, with the associated sensations and feelings, to another unknown place.*

The pace of our therapeutic encounter was *slow and steady* and I would have been aware of the need for this to be so from the cues in Liz's body language. There were felt moments of *calm serenity* in which we were both caught up as I empathised with what Liz was feeling. Also, the particular nuances of Liz's own early experience would have been enhanced by the sound of the gentle female voice of the singer which perhaps linked with the trace of mother's/grandmother's voice deep in implicit memory. Through attentive listening we were both caught up in this musical experience affecting both our mind/brain.

As has been noted above, the music in our shared experience of listening could have held the dynamic aspects of Liz's mother and grandmother in the transference and counter-transference. Although we both had strong feelings in response to the music I was aware of the need to listen to my own feelings and put them to one side while I empathised with Liz's feelings. I was there for her, she was not there for me.

In the spoken narrative in this session we explored what might have been her early experience all those years ago in attachment to her mother and grandmother. She herself linked the Angel aria to the experience of being born and the 'time immediately afterwards'. There was anxiety in the room at this point. Liz's feared experience of the unknown could have been evoked by the singing voice of Gerontius who expresses fear and terror of the unknown on his journey to God and is soothed by the Angel's voice. It was important to hold Liz here in a symbolic manner through how I made eye contact with her and how I responded with my voice. It would not be therapeutic or right for Liz to be re-traumatized again by me as she had been in the pain clinic. Wilkinson writes on the therapeutic technique of drawing back from such a destructive inner process:

> 'Often it may help to begin to slow one's speech, to use a calm voice, often with a lower tone, speaking in what Williams has described as "pastel rather than primary colours". It may be that the therapist will make eye contact in what I can only describe as a "holding" sort of way. The aim is not reassurance *per se*, or avoidance of the emerging material, but rather to enable the patient to remain "in mind" and able to work.'[6]

Liz later wrote about this session and one interpretation of her writing could be that she seems to reflect on very early experiences associated unconsciously with the time of her birth. Liz could not have remembered anything explicitly about this early time but the feelings and sensations she describes could have been resonating with it.

She writes of her feelings of being weightless . . . 'a bit like lying in a swimming pool, just relaxed in the warm water with the sound wrapped all around me like a blanket'. Liz next goes on to link the Angel aria to the great Amen chorus at the end of the *Messiah* by Handel. She writes:

> 'My breathing changes and becomes increased and shallower and my heart rate rises so that I begin to feel the pulse in my neck and right in my ears. If the music becomes more exciting my skin begins to tingle and the sound if loud enough feels as if everything is blown out of my head . . . and I am completely somewhere else on a "high" that I cannot explain.'

It is of note that Liz wrote this reflection at home and not in the consulting room with me. However, she has managed to regulate the excitement well in that she has written it down. It has come into words. Fonagy writes:

> 'The ability to represent the idea of an affect is crucial in the achievement of control over overwhelming affect.'[7]

The next piece of music Liz brought in on 18 August was the *Queen Symphony* by Tolga Kashif.

The *Queen Symphony* by Tolga Kashif

In the *Queen Symphony* by Tolga Kashif, Liz was most aware of feelings of joy and sorrow experienced at the same time and that the ending had great importance. This joy and sorrow, although held in the music, could be said to have come together in a more grounded way than that of the previous music. This was demonstrated by Liz's choice of the *Queen Symphony*, which she associated with a real live human being and not an angel.

In Liz's life, her grandmother, who reminded her of the old Queen Mary, had a big influence on Liz and part of the sorrow would have been that she could not always be with her. The joy and sorrow seemed to become more articulated in her own life during this session and the other world which she wanted to escape to might have been a 'heaven' where her grandmother would be with her all the time.

Analysis of the shared listening experience

In this music the *pulse* is more alive and energetic, as was our conversation. The *quality* or flow of the music was more varied and alive. Musical leaps of exuberance and freedom contributed to this liveliness. The *narrative* of the words set to music is to do with living your own life with enthusiasm, especially in the song *Who Wants to Live Forever?*.

There was an uneasy feel about the quality of the exuberant melodic leaps linked to the idea of dying, in the song *Who Wants to Live Forever?*. The narrative of this passage might have resonated with the story of her grandmother who was strong and determined and trod her own pathway in life (the pulse of her way of living), but died when Liz was 11.

Liz was aware of key changes, which seem to have a significant effect on her. She writes:

> 'Near the end there are two moments when a key change in the music twists the intensity so much that I feel this within my body to the extent that I begin to shudder. This music is rich in sound and emotion and seems to get right into the very core of me.'

This bringing into words of Liz's experience of being with grandma and the pain of heartbreak and feelings of loss in relation to her in her early years had been worked with in the previous session. Listening to this music in particular might have been a further example of active connections between left and right hemispheres in the brain, the plasticity that enables change to occur. Wilkinson writes that:

> 'Exchanges that involve putting feelings into words encourage healthy and integrated functioning of both hemispheres of the brain and are an intrinsic part of the process on coming into mind.'[8]

The next piece of music chosen was the first movement of Dvorak's *Second Symphony*. This was the first piece of music that she connected with her mother. With it came lots of memories of her mother and father caring for her.

Dvorak's *Second Symphony* – the first movement

In the passage from the first movement chosen by Liz the *pulse* of the music is measured and flowing, and a descending melodic line has the *quality* of a caressing gesture. It has a relaxed flow and is almost hesitant. The *narrative* of the music is abstract in that there is no story originally attached to the music but as Liz remembers, this passage was used to introduce the Charles Dickens story of *Nicholas Nickleby* on the radio.

As we spoke about what it meant for Liz, the *pulse* of our conversation became less continuous in that the flow and *quality* of our engagement was broken by silences as she began to recall some warm memories of her mother writing to the BBC about the music and buying a record of it for her. This ushered in more warm *narrative* of explicit memories of her parents and her grandmother who had died just before her 11th birthday.

Analysis of the shared listening

After listening to the musical passage our words together were gentle and Liz's voice was softer than usual and became hesitant. Our conversation had a caring *quality* about it and this led to a caring quality in Liz's *narrative* in which she spoke about the atmosphere in her parents' home, with the warm colours which she is now using to redecorate her own home. She noted that her choice of lighting in her newly decorated room reminded her of the soft gas lamps in her grandmother's house. A very rich narrative followed about her grandmother's life and it felt in the room as if she was really grieving for this much loved and admired woman.

But this was followed by the *first* warm memory of her mother and sitting close to her on the bus and remembering the colours and texture of her dress. This gentle passage of music seemed very important in that Liz's experience of it became linked to visual and tactile recall now articulated in words, that is, in explicit memory. She remembered verbally the warm colours in her grandmother's home that she now deliberately uses in the redecoration of her own home. She then recalled the diamond patterning and the texture of her mother's dress, which are echoed in the diamond patterning and colours of her new wallpaper.

When I asked Liz what she understood about what might be happening through our working with music, she replied that she was discovering pleasant memories but that the feelings of loss were still there.

'Come ye Daughters Share my Mourning' from the *St Matthew Passion*

Before Liz brought in the next piece of music on 19 January 2004 she had painted a beautiful garden scene with buddleia and butterflies, which we enjoyed at the start of the session. I silently associated this painting with her grandmother but waited to see if she had brought in more music. Liz presented a passage from the *St Matthew Passion* by Bach, 'Come ye Daughters Share my Mourning'. She herself writes of the *pulse, quality* and *narrative* in this music and in her experience. This was a surprising development and not discussed between us at all.

> 'There is a strong pulse beat and I am aware of the flowing crotchet/quaver rhythm in the bass line. We have 16 bars introduction and then the chorus comes in "Come ye Daughters, Share my Mourning". This is so beautiful it makes my toes curl. The sound fills my body and head and for a few seconds blasts out all the stuff in there which seems to drag me down. There is a build up in the orchestra and then we get to the tune. Such beautiful words and a lovely line to sing which goes on until the end of the movement. The final chord completely enthrals me.'

Trevarthen writes of this kind of feeling story:

> 'Music does more than please us. It gives us an experience unfolding, a narrative without reference that feels important.'[9]

It certainly felt important for Liz in the counter-transference but she was unaware, as I was, of what the particular relevance and importance this music had for her at this stage. It could have been that for Liz there was as yet no explicit connection to her own grief. The women grieving, and 'daughters' in particular, did not seem to be 'in mind' and resonate with her own grieving. It could also have been signalling that some time soon her intense grief might be coming to an end. This feeling of solace was in the room in symbolic form.

The realisation that she was a daughter to her mother, and may have been for a short time like a daughter when she was cared for by grandmother, was not mentioned at this stage. There did not seem to be an explicit connection encoded in words between her own experience of grief and that of the mothers and daughters whose experience of grief and solace we were listening to. This could be because the feeling traces of her own grief were still held in implicit memory, that is, encoded very early in her right brain/mind before the age of three.

However, in the process of working through her feelings about this music Liz brought in a further painting of a lonely seascape, which she showed me alongside the buddleia and butterfly painting. Perhaps here we were experiencing the memory traces of being with her mother and grandmother in the room. The lonely seascape could have belonged to the early feelings and sensations associated with her mother and the buddleia picture associated with her grandmother. It could be that these traces in the brain were now framed on paper and perhaps more connected with the left brain than before.

Having revisited her sorrow in the room with me, Liz then decided to write her poem *My Returning Journey*. Here she had moved to another position in that she was reflecting on her present inner mental state not in painting but in words. There was now a real process of right/left brain integration taking place.

Analysis of the shared listening experience

This way of listening to music within the consulting room engages in particular with right brain feeling responses. When these responses, which were originally held in music for Liz, move to painting and then into words, it is now understood that new left brain connections are being made. Cozolino writes on this process in the brain as follows:

> [It is] 'the blending of the strengths of the right and left hemisphere that allows for the maximum integration of our cognitive and emotional experience with our inner and outer worlds.'[10]

It is suggested here that, through this process of Liz and I actively listening to music together and then through the enjoyment of her artwork and poetry within psychodynamic psychotherapy, Liz was integrating more of her early loving experiences. She was beginning not only to feel and sense the traces of the positive and loving aspects of her early attachment experience, but she was now bringing later loving experiences more fully to mind. The vitality of the feelings and sensations, which had been held in implicit memory and previously unavailable in words, was very present in the room and articulated verbally. It could be that new neural pathways were being built. It could be that Teicher is referring to this process when he writes:

> 'Perhaps as yet speculative, nevertheless it may be inferred that the therapeutic process and the evolving symbolizations associated with it can develop new neural pathways in the brain, and in particular can develop the fibre tract known as the corpus callosum that is the major highway between the two hemispheres, shown to be reduced through the effects of trauma.'[11]

This process continued with the next piece of music, 'The White Tree' from the film music *The Return of the King*.

'The White Tree' from the film music *The Return of the King*

Again Liz wrote at length about her experience in terms of *pulse*, *quality* and *narrative*. (The words in parenthesis are the author's.) She writes:

> 'What I remember best was what was happening in my body. The movement starts quietly with strings playing. This makes me feel calm (quality). The tempo then changes and I can feel my breathing changing. The *pulse* in the music becomes more insistent and I seem to be waiting for the repeated

theme to come. Each time the main chord changes it moves the music on, driving it forward; building up a tremendous crescendo. My breathing changes, my heart quickens, I cannot sit still. I want to conduct, count, physically feel the beat. There is a dramatic moment when every instrument, the strings, the brass, get faster and faster, until the moment of climax, when all the instruments along with gongs and percussion stop. At this moment I feel release, like set free to fly (emotional narrative).'

I would suggest that this is a very articulate description of Malloch's categories of *communicative musicality*. It could be said that we are also witnessing the Intrinsic Motive Pulse (IMP) now very active in Liz and enabling this sophisticated verbal communication.

Trevarthen writes of how:

'All our explorations of the musicality of an infant's life in human company confirm the idea that free and sympathetic expression of what we call Intrinsic Motive Pulse (IMP) of moving and feeling is necessary for the development of the mind and for emotional health. That is why musical communication (with children and adults) can be such powerful therapy.'[12]

Analysis of the shared listening experience

When Liz and I spoke on 15 March 2004 about her poem and the music 'The White Tree', Liz commented that it was 'about movement and becoming alive – like a bird flying, soaring'.

At this point in the therapy it seemed that Liz had now reached a position where she felt sufficiently free within her psyche to find a space in her mind where the experience of joy was possible. To use Trevarthen's phrase, through music Liz's IMP for her expression of movement and feeling was now freed up in a way not available to her adult self-in-relation before therapy. This IMP with which we come into the world 'moves the body and also excites the neurochemistry of felt elation and sadness, or of vitality and repose'. Trevarthen continues:

'As soon as music is made, by singing or playing, or even vividly "hearing" it in the mind, the pulse and emotional variation of movement is back in charge, proving that it was present all along, unconsciously, in the architecture of the brain's trace of music.'[13]

Liz's verbal description of her active listening experience of the music 'The White Tree' had a new liveliness and animation about it, which supports Trevarthen's writing. This sense of freedom and confidence was again noted on 25 April when she described hearing the Litolff *Piano Concerto*. This again might have been an instance of right-brain-to-right-brain communication between us. I hadn't heard the piece that morning nor did I know it was going to be performed, but her liveliness and sparkle as she described the pianist's playing brought the name of this particular piece to my mind. This was a happy 'co-incidence' shared.

Our work ended on 22 June and Liz wanted to write about where she was now.

Here Liz writes about listening to music in a different way. She is more aware of her physical sensations and in particular she is aware of the flow of music as it connects with sadness and also with joy. Liz now writes that she experiences the 'full circle of feelings, a richer experience', but not only are these experiences *in the music* but *in my own head and body*. Much has come together for Liz.

There is, however, a further postscript. Liz wrote and told me that she had written a further poem and enquired if it might be useful for the book. I am reminded on reading it of Frank Lake's phrase that there is improvement and a measure of cure when 'You have *it* (the depression, pain and grief) and *it* no longer has you'.[14] Liz's poem follows.

My Journey Onward

Blue sky, clouds white and fluffy
Birds singing, swifts screaming
Smiling faces, joyful laughter
People round me, laughing with me.

Back behind me dark and dingy
Black tunnel still awaits me
Can feel its pull, can see the darkness
Conscious of its ever presence.

I look around me to the distance
Life's companions now around me
Family and friends join with me
On my journey onward.

If I feel; the tunnel beckoning
Drawing me towards its darkness
My eyes look out
Remembering those who love me
And the people who have helped me
Realise now it's them, and prayer and music
Bringing me the peace I've always needed.

Liz: 6 March 2006

References

1 Malloch S (1999) Mothers and infants and communicative musicality. *Musicae Scientiae (Special Issue 1999–2000).* The European Society for Cognitive Sciences, Belgium, pp. 29–57.
2 Nocker-Ribaupierre M (ed.) *Music Therapy for Premature and Newborn Infants* Barcelona Publishers, Gilsum NH, pp. 97–113.
3 Ibid, pp. 97–8.
4 Ibid, p. 98.
5 Trevarthen C (2006) *Wie schreibt die Autobiographie eines Kindes. Warum*

Menschen Sich Erinnern Können. (Fortschritte der Interdisziplinaren Gedashtnish-forschung). Hrsg. Hans Markowitsch and Harald Weltzer. Klett-Cotta, Stuttgart, pp. 225–55. (Translation Karoline Tschuggnall).

6 Wilkinson M (2006) *Coming into Mind.* Routledge, London and New York, p. 80.

7 Fonagy P (1991) Thinking about thinking: some clinical and theoretical considerations in the treatment of a borderline patient. *International Journal of Psychoanalysis.* **76**: 639–56. Quoted in M Wilkinson (2006) *Coming into Mind.* Routledge, London and New York, p. 94.

8 Wilkinson M (2006) *Coming into Mind.* Routledge, London and New York, p. 113.

9 Trevarthen C and Malloch S (2002) The musical lives of babies and families. *Journal of Zero to Three: National Centre for Infants, Toddlers and Families.* **23** (1): 12.

10 Cozolino L (2002) *The Neuroscience of Psychotherapy.* WW Norton and Co., New York and London, p. 115. Quoted in M Wilkinson (2006) *Coming into Mind.* Routledge, London and New York, p. 12.

11 Teicher M (2000) Wounds that time won't heal: The neurobiology of child abuse. *Cerebrum.* **2**(4). Quoted in M Wilkinson (2006) *Coming into Mind.* Routledge, London and New York, p. 11.

12 Trevarthen C and Malloch S (2002) The musical lives of babies and families. *Journal of Zero to Three: National Centre for Infants, Toddlers and Families.* **23** (1): 16.

13 Trevarthen C (1999) Musicality and the intrinsic motive pulse: evidence from human psychobiology and infant communication. *Musicae Scientiae (Special Issue 1999–2000).* The European Society for Cognitive Sciences, Belgium, pp. 7–8.

14 Frank Lake (1914–1982) Founder of Clinical Theology. Personal communication.

CHAPTER 13

Where are we now?

To throw more light on the music chosen by patients within psychotherapy we explored, at the beginning of this book, what music meant for four people in the public eye. We discovered that their choices of music were not only very different from each other in genre, but that what the important music of their choice meant for them was also very different. We then reflected on what this might be about. We reached the conclusion that each interviewee had a very different experience of music because of the culture into which they had been born and further to this they would each would have been affected by the vagaries of their life experiences. However, we discovered that, although they were each individual persons, there were aspects of their listening to music that were similar. For example, music enlivened their lives and made their living in relationship with other persons more interesting.

Mercedes Pavlicevic's life's work is about engaging in a therapeutic way with persons through musical improvisation. Her therapeutic method puts them and her in touch with human energy, the spark of life, and she does this through playing and improvising music with them and understanding the shared process of communicative musicality. This leads them to a better psychological place as persons living in relationship in the world. In Katie Melua's interview she spoke of how her life is concerned with singing and creating songs. This enlivens her being and she has this effect on many audiences of listeners throughout the world. For Baroness Neuberger music means a reflection of the order she seeks in her own busy life as she works to contribute to the welfare of others from a religious and political stance. For Benjamin Zephaniah the rhythm and move-ment in music mirrors being alive itself and the dignity of being human. This he communicates to a wider audience of listeners through his poetry, his music and his communicative musicality. These interviewees, however, were not talking with me in the context or 'habitus' of psychotherapy where, over time, the relationship with the therapist inevitably colours what the patient chooses and needs to hear within therapy.

We next considered some philosophical theories which were near to the experience of music and found a strand of philosophical thought starting with Zuckerkandl's idea of music as outside the experience of the person but relating through the 'motion in the dynamic field of tones'. Langer's thinking moved to a much more inward understanding of music in that she understands it as a symbol of the internal world of feeling and we gained insight into this internal

165

world through listening to music. Cumming's view was that understanding a piece of music emotionally is like getting to know someone's special mood or way of being. These philosophical theories placed listening to music both within the person and outside the person.

Then we considered 'everyday' music and noted De Nora's, Sloboda's and Juslin's work on identifying the difference between 'everyday' music and 'special music'. But listening to music within psychotherapy would seem to cut across this boundary of difference between the 'everyday' and the 'special' in that the patient's shared experience of listening to music is central to listening to music together. In this sense each passage of music that the patient brings into the consulting room is special.

The context of the experience of listening to music came to the fore on considering the work of Judith Becker. She challenged the single brain approach to traditional scientific research on the experience of music and introduced the concept of the 'habitus' of music which is:

> 'Complex systems of thought and behaviour concerning what music means, what it is for, how it is perceived and what might be appropriate expressive responses.'[1]

This idea of the 'habitus' of listening to music was found to be helpful in clearly identifying what needed to be thought about in the shared experience of listening to music with the patient. The patient was not listening to music alone in that this is a special shared experience. We are both involved as adult persons in this therapeutic experience.

We then turned to music therapy and what we might learn from Guided Imagery and Music (GIM) and Regulative Music Therapy. Their focus on the programme of music itself chosen by the therapist or in conversation with the therapist did not seem to sit easily with the shared listening experience in psychotherapy as described in this book. Also, the relationship with the patient is understood as separate from the shared musical experience in the consulting room.

However, Isabelle Frohne-Hagemann's thinking on a musical gestalt is particularly interesting, and also her ideas on there being a hierarchy in mixed modal therapy starting with movement and hearing and developing through sight and then speech are particularly important. This developmental progress resonated with the work done with Liz where she was able to communicate in prose and poetry her experiences of listening to music in psychotherapy. We briefly noted musicology's current interest in the experiencing listener and music. Papers written on Jung's 'collective unconscious' and listening to music is of particular interest. It is hoped that this experiential strand of persons listening to music within the discipline of musicology will further grow and develop outside as well as inside America, Russia and Canada.

The experience of the musical origins of self-in-relationship was then considered through the work of Trevarthen and Malloch and 'communicative musicality' was explored. In infancy 'communicative musicality' is first found in the non-verbal and pre-verbal joyous meeting and engagement between infants and mothers or infants and first carers. As adults, when we move by clapping our hands at a concert in appreciation, we are showing our 'communicative musicality'. What is most interesting in this twenty-first century is that the movement of jumping up and down and arm waving at a pop concert is also a form of communicative musicality. It could be said that communicative musicality lies somewhere between the person and the discipline of music. It is physical movement and appreciative gesture in the sonic space between the performer and listener. It is not entirely of the person in that they are performing or responding to music or a musical sound, nor is it entirely of music. Music cannot exist without persons at some point. Communicative musicality flows in the human experience of music between persons.

Liz's experience of listening to music within psychotherapy was then described and reflected upon. Although we examined in some detail her choices of music and what these choices meant for her within the therapeutic engagement, we did not consider her aesthetic responses at that time. Ellen Dissanayake's thinking on 'natural aesthetics' outlined in Chapter 5 would seem to come nearest Liz's experience of listening to music and especially within psychotherapy.

Liz's natural aesthetics

In Dissanayake's 'natural aesthetics' the first criterion with regards to quality was that any choice of music should be accessible and striking in some way and all Liz's choices met this first criterion. The second criterion in addition to the first, was tangible relevance. This again was met in that each of Liz's choices had tangible relevance and particular meaning for her. The third criterion of evocative resonance for the listener was described by Dissanayake as the experience of the music having 'more than meets the eye' about it. This was certainly the case in Liz's experience of listening to music within psychotherapy in the consulting room. This 'more than meets the eye' referred to the complexity or density of meaning the work has for the listener. This complexity and density of meaning for Liz was considered more fully in the description of the therapeutic work and her own written account of what music meant for her as she progressed through the therapy. She described how she was able to move through different states of feeling associated with difficult periods in her life. But where does this leave us? We still do not have a model of mind to which we can turn, in order to systematically explore and begin to understand more about the experience of music within psychotherapy and how to describe it in a thought-out way.

Towards a model of mind of music in psychotherapy

It is not surprising that we as yet do not have such a model of mind. Such an inter-subjective model of the experience of listening to music based on inter-disciplinary thinking would need to recognise and give appropriate importance to music in our lives as a living symbol of who we are in relationship and not consider it only as entertainment. This model of mind/brain/body is not yet available in the current literature. However, there are important advances in the thinking and practice of modern attachment theory and, along with under-standings in affective neuroscience and advances in musicology, psychotherapy with music and GIM would seem to offer the possibility of a future integrative therapeutic theory. This future integrative therapeutic theory might well encompass listening to music in the consulting room. In particular, attachment theory rooted in infant–carer communication, and communicative musicality before the emergence in the infant of cognitive thought, would be a rich arena for information exchange towards such a theory. The ground work for such an exchange of pre-verbal or non-verbal research has been laid down by Allan Schore who writes that when we speak or write of a self we are really referring to a self-in-relationship. He writes:

> 'There is widespread agreement that the brain is a self-organizing system, but there is perhaps less of an appreciation of the fact that the self-organizing of the developing brain occurs in the context of a relationship with another self, another brain.'[2]

When it comes to the beginnings of who we are as babies and infants and how we begin to communicate and further establish our selves-in-relationship with our first carers through musical behaviours in mind/brain/body, Trevarthen's and Malloch's work on communicative musicality is important. Their writing is a scientific measurable developmental contribution to a proposed interdisciplin-ary model of mind, as it dovetails comfortably with psychoanalytic theory and practice in the form of modern attachment theory. As the infant experience in early life is multimodal in character, other arts research could be incorporated. In particular, Trevarthen and Malloch's work on infant–mother communica-tive musicality is held to be the vehicle through which not only secure infant–mother attachment is expressed and observed but it is also the main motive for cultural learning in the infant. Writing on pride and shame, two of the powerful emotions associated with companionship. Trevarthen states:

> 'These emotions of companionship (pride and shame) are very important in the development of happy self-confidence, at any age . . . Our evidence shows that the baby has a well-integrated self at birth, an effective self. But it has to work out what to do with this motivated life it has, and one of the first things to learn is the meaning of the world: to learn the meaning of other older persons' actions . . . The meaning of the world can only be acquired in

communication and collaboration with other people. There is no such thing as meaning found entirely by a single self.'[3]

In this context, cultural learning not only means that the infant needs to become at ease in the culture of becoming a person-in-relationship with mother or others within the same human society or grouping but it also means the infant becoming slowly aware of what is to be strived for. This would be a sense of quality in the arts of that particular culture. They would learn what is considered to be fine and of quality in music, dance, painting, sculpture, etc., an aesthetic mode of being in the world. This recognition of the need for the presence of another self and how necessary this is as a motive for cultural learning has also been noted in the writing of Judith Becker and the 'habitus' of listening to music and Ellen Dissanayake in her 'natural aesthetics'.

The origin of aesthetic experience in the infant mind

But where might we now position ourselves aesthetically in the practice of listening to music in psychotherapy with the patient in the consulting room? We have pointed to Trevarthen and Malloch's work from the discipline of neuroscience on infant–mother communicative musicality which encompasses the inner and outer experiences of moving sympathetically with one another and the musical vocal and aural sounds between them. We have also considered the first aesthetic moments in understandings of the infant/mother being together as described by Trevarthen and Malloch.

However, Bollas, from a psychoanalytic perspective, suggests that our important experiences of music will have a trace in the brain of this early infant–carer aesthetic[4] and Winnicott's idea of the baby not being a single self but a self-in-relationship is near Bollas' thinking here.[5] Further to this, the idea that the infant does not thrive as a single self but as a self-in-relationship is echoed by the writing of Schore on attachment and developmentally-oriented psychoanalytic psychotherapy.[6]

But is there any evidence of a comfortable welcome for the practice of listening to music chosen by the patient in the world of the talking therapies? This practice links Trevarthen and Malloch's work with Bollas on the first aesthetic as it appears in adult aesthetic experience of listening to music chosen by the patient within psychotherapy.

Music talked about in psychotherapy

Lachmann's writing seems to offer a home for this kind of thinking and practice of listening to music within the consulting room in his paper 'Words and Music'. Here he describes how a patient might describe the experience of music in words.[7] It is thought about and discussed in the consulting room and an outline of what music is in terms of tonality and rhythm and the inner psychological categories of experience are named.

For example, Kohut's 1950s libido theory of sexuality is understood as the discharge of tension and release and is discussed in relation to the tension and release in the rhythmic and tonal flow in music. He then turns to the function of the analyst listening to the patient's voice. This is linked to listening to the patient's 'music', that is, the music or flow beneath the words. As the paper continues it becomes clear that music is being discussed as if it existed alongside the person, and the inner individual experience of shared music in the consulting room remains untouched. Music itself is *not* brought into the room.

This position changes subtly with a description of studies by Beatrice Beebe *et al.*[8] on the place of vocal rhythm co-ordination between adult pairs and between infants and adults. One interesting finding for psychotherapy is that 'Adult partners in a conversation tend to co-ordinate with each other's vocal rhythm' also 'Co-ordinating one's own vocal timing with that of a partner, whether infant or adult, is crucial for the infant's social development as well as for adult relationships.' These findings seem to dovetail with Trevarthen's work on communicative musicality, but we seem to be no nearer to understanding the shared aesthetic experience of music nor the possibility of accepting the experience of listening to music within the consulting room as part of the therapeutic relationship. Here one might ask why is this so?

Reflecting on the paper by Lachmann, it is noted that it is called 'Words and Music' – a clear separation between verbal language and music, so we are no further forward in finding a home in which to situate the practice of listening to music within psychotherapy. However, one interviewee, Katie Melua, was aware that music was like the 'sound track' to her emotional life and that could be said to be describing a clear separation psychologically. She was regarding music as an outside phenomenon at this point, just as Lachmann does. When she sings, however, she is very much within the music as well as being outside it. She is a performer, a listener and a creative artist. It is a feature of her artistry that she can manage this intermediate place between inner and outer experience with ease. This point of view would seem to support Winnicott's (1971) theory of creativity. In this creative place he writes that:

> 'No longer are we either introvert or extrovert. We experience life in the area of transitional phenomena, in the exciting interweave of subjectivity and objective observation, and in an area that is intermediate between the inner reality of the individual and the shared reality of the world that is external to individuals.'[9]

However, Katie was not the only one of our interviewees who was able for periods of time to inhabit this inner and outer reality. They each had this ability to live in the inner and outer worlds with comparative ease, and music and/or poetry was the place where this inner and outer experience was lived out. The point made here is that this position of occupying inner and outer psychological space at the same time is a commonly held position of being human.

Inner and outer reality in the consulting room

Following on from Dissanayake's theory of 'natural aesthetics', listening to the patient's music in the consulting room, these special passages of music would be called aesthetic moments. If this is so, allowing music to come into the consulting room would be giving permission for these important aesthetic moments to be re-experienced and shared with another human being. When these aesthetic moments occur in the consulting room both therapist and patient are involved in listening to a passage of music chosen by the patient. The passage of music however has only ever lasted for two or three minutes at the most in my experience. The choice of whether to bring in a passage of music or not would be in the entire control of the patient who can make a cognitive choice. If they are unsure then they simply won't bring it into the room. Theoretically, when the relationship within therapy feels safe enough, or to put it differently, the patient's ego-strength in relation to the therapist feels safe and secure enough, they will be able to make a choice about this. Until this point is reached in psychotherapy and the patient declares that he or she is going to introduce music into the room, the usual verbal exchanges or intermittent verbal exchanges would be observed.

The aural shadow of the object

It seems, however, that patients choose to bring music into the therapy when there are no longer words to frame what they want to communicate. I am reminded here of Antonia Murphy's patient and also Fiona Aitken's patient described in the Coda (*see* Chapter 14).

However, when words are not available to the patient it is often understood by the therapist as resistance and the patient is said to be angry with the therapist. This may be so and possible ways in which the patient might be angry would need to be explored. But this so called anger might also be a hopeless frustration that something non-verbal of them is not being heard and attended to. This again could be interpreted as the reality of life in that 'the mother'/therapist must indeed frustrate the infant and not gratify this early infantile need. This would also need to be considered. But there is another possible explanation for the patient's silence, the quality of which would need to be identified by the therapist in the counter-transference.

It could be that in this non-verbal place in the consulting room, there is a silent emptiness. It may need to be considered that there is a requirement for that empty space to be filled by a loving meeting in a symbolic mode experienced by both patient and therapist. This kind of emptiness may be the patient's search for a 'transformational object' the trace of which lies within a very early non-verbal experience in relation to the patient's first carer.[10] It could also be argued that this kind of experience might never really have happened for the patient and this is what they are trying to *create* with the therapist. But there is truth in Winnicott's idea that the patient just would not have survived emotionally if there had not been some trace experience of warm intimacy as a reality.

In the consulting room this feeling state of silent emptiness and loss of human contact cannot be verbalised because, as has been said in an earlier chapter when an experience has been encoded in one form it is very difficult to meet with it in therapy in another. It may be therefore that music fills that space of silent emptiness for the patient and that is why they need to hear it in the presence of the therapist who makes this experience human. Listening to music within psychotherapy enhances the experience of self-in-relationship for the patient. But why does music need to be brought into the consulting room? Why can't the patient just listen to the music they need to listen to at home?

The answers to these questions must lie in the notion that the presence of human beings is necessary for this kind of lasting transformation of the patient's self-in-relationship. The arts alone are not sufficient to repair early relational trauma. They can temporarily soothe and assuage it but it is persons-in-relationship through the therapeutic medium of music which ushers in more lasting change.

The emptiness that the patient feels may not only be the absence of the beauty and/or liveliness of the lost aesthetic moment which was not repeated enough to be sculpted into the formation of the brain/mind, it might also perhaps be a felt experience of the absence of human flesh and blood. Bollas writes:

> 'Society cannot possibly meet the requirements of the subject, as the mother met the needs of the infant, but in the arts we have a location for such occasional recollections: intense memories of the process of self-transformation.'[11]

However, Bollas is writing of the arts alongside the process of psychotherapy, not within it. When the patient experiences this state outside the consulting room, this emptiness is assuaged by listening to music because there are flowing sounds which provide an aural image of a warm human feeling. This is perhaps the trace memory of the first aesthetic of being-in-relationship with the first carer or carers evoked by the relations between the tones, and the safety and security of the music having a beginning, middle and end – a gestalt of being-in-relationship. Bollas writes:

> 'The mother's idiom of care and the infant's experience of this handling is born of the first if not the earliest human aesthetic. It is the most profound occasion when the nature of the self is formed and transformed by the environment. The uncanny pleasure of being held by a poem, a composition, a painting or, for that matter, any object rests on those moments when the infant's internal world is partly given form by the mother since he cannot shape them or link them together without her coverage.' He continues, 'Each

aesthetic experience is transformational . . . so the search for the aesthetic object is a quest for the transformational object.'[12]

When the patient brings music into the consulting room, they are searching in part perhaps for a transformational object which they have experienced briefly but then lost. As has been noted above, as an adult patient, listening to music itself will transform his being in the world for a few brief minutes but the sense of loss returns – loss of feeling good and loss of company with another human being. As the therapist witnesses the aesthetic experience of the patient listening to a passage of music in the consulting room, the therapist is permitted to be in the patient's aesthetic space. Because of the therapist's empathic stance they are able to be with the patient in a special shared intimacy through the medium of music. Over a period of time there is right-brain to right-brain communication within the therapeutic relationship and a more lasting element of transformation seems to occur than with the patient listening to music alone.

When the music ceases to sound the patient 'knows' that the therapist, another human being, has occupied that intense non-verbal momentarily symbiotic dynamic sounding space with them. They know yet again, and perhaps repeatedly that they are not alone and without human contact of this special intensity when they needed it, and this loss has been 'heard' and experienced with another human being in the room.

In the earliest aesthetic, Bollas writes that the intensity of the experience was able to be felt by the infant because they were psychically 'covered by mother'.[13] In the consulting room the empathy and attention to the patient by the therapist symbolically covers the patient during the perhaps intense arousal of the aesthetic experience. Also the frame of the music, the form which provides it with an experiential beginning, middle and end also holds the patient. Bollas writes:

> 'I believe that if we investigate many types of object relating we will discover that the subject is seeking the transformational object and aspiring to be matched in symbiotic harmony within an aesthetic frame that promises to metamorphose the self.'[14]

Bollas here was writing as an analyst and would not as I understand it have listened to music with the patient. But his writing on what is required when the patient is in need of ego transformation is to be noted when working with patients and music in the consulting room. He writes:

> 'What is needed is an initial experience of successive ego transformations that are identified with the analyst and the analytic process. In such moments, the patient experiences interpretations primarily for their capacity to match his internal mood, feeling or thought, and such moments of rapport lead the patient to "re-experience", the transformational object relation.'[15]

This writing along with what we now know about neural pathways in the brain and neural connectivity may begin to explain the longer lasting transformation of the self-in-relationship described above with Liz. Wilkinson writes:

'One speculates that in the consulting room through the revisiting of experiences that went to establish attachment in the first year of life, new neural pathways and patterns of connectivity in the right hemisphere of the brain may be established. Communication between the hemispheres means that experience can then be put into words and processed by the left.'[16]

Liz's writing and her ability to reflect on her experience of music and put it into words would be evidence of a transformative experience of who she was as a person-in-relationship in the world. Not all aesthetic moments are of such intensity but they will all have arisen from our first aesthetic with our mother or first carer and will carry the trace of this experience in all our later aesthetic experiences. Our chosen music, music that is important for us whether in therapy or in life in general, will bear the trace of this early aesthetic experience. Perhaps there is a place for listening to music within the psychological therapies. Bollas writing 20 years ago on the arts and their relation to the non-verbal ways of being in the world is heard here as sounding an encouraging note. He writes:

'I am sure that psychoanalysts could learn a great deal about this form of knowing from modern dance where the dancer expresses the unthought known through body knowledge. And it may well be that musical representation is somewhere between the unthought known and thought proper.'[17]

Between the 'unthought known' and 'thought proper' is exactly where listening to music chosen by the patient is situated. More research is needed to bring it into 'thought proper', but always leaving a portal open for the 'unthought known'.

References

1 Becker J (2001) Anthropological perspectives on music and emotion. In: P Juslin and J Sloboda (eds) *Music and Emotion*. Oxford University Press, Oxford, p. 137.
2 Schore A (2003) The human unconscious: the development of the right brain and its role in early emotional life. In: V Green (ed.) *Emotional Development in Psychoanalysis, Attachment Theory and Neuroscience*. Brunner-Routledge, Hove and New York, p. 23.
3 Trevarthen C (2003) Neuroscience and intrinsic psychodynamics: current knowledge and potential for therapy. In: J Corrigall and H Wilkinson (eds) *Revolutionary Connections*. Karnac Books, London, p. 67.
4 Bollas C (1987) *The Shadow of the Object*. Columbia University Press, New York, p. 14.
5 Winnicott DW (1990) Parent–infant relationship. In: *The Maturational Processes and the Facilitating Environment*. Karnac Books, London, p. 39.
6 Schore A (2003) The human unconscious: the development of the right brain and its role in early emotional life. In: V Green (ed.) *Emotional Development in Psychoanalysis, Attachment Theory and Neuroscience*. Brunner-Routledge, Hove and New York, pp. 23–54.

7   Lachmann F (2001) Words and music. *Progress in Self Psychology*. Volume 17.
8   Ibid, p. 3.
9   Winnicott DW (1988) (First published 1971). *Playing and Reality*. Penguin Books, p. 75.
10 Bollas C (1987) *The Shadow of the Object*. Columbia University Press, New York, p. 14.
11 Ibid, p. 29.
12 Ibid, p. 33.
13 Ibid, p. 32.
14 Ibid, p. 40.
15 Ibid, p. 23.
16 Wilkinson M (2006) *Coming into Mind*. Routledge, London and New York, p. 30.
17 Bollas C (1987) *The Shadow of the Object*. Columbia University Press, New York, p. 282.

CHAPTER 14

Coda

When music comes into the room

Psychotherapists Antonia Murphy and Fiona Aitken have both had patients bring music into the consulting room. At the time they did not experience the music in the room but listened to it afterwards. What follows are their accounts of these experiences. It seems important that if music is to be brought into the room and heard there, this must be agreed early-on in the therapy so that the therapist is not taken unawares.

Antonia Murphy

About four years into his psychotherapy R spoke of a song he kept hearing on the radio that he had bought for himself. It was a pop song. In the session that day he told me 'Every time I play this song I think of you.' Next session he handed me a cassette tape saying, 'I wanted you to hear it . . . you can have this'. It seemed very important for R that he was able to give me the song and that I should hear it too as yet I had no idea of its content.

R was a deeply damaged man in his mid 30s when he began weekly therapy with me. He was a younger child in an impoverished family. His father had died when he was eight years old and his mother had seemingly singled him out to be the family's hit man. Any trouble in the family and R was the culprit. But any trouble outside and R was sent to sort it out. Mother neglected to love him and at the same time made use of him; violence and putting the fear of God into anyone and everyone became second nature to him. He was a very successful thug because he rarely had to hit anyone, he was so menacing. R had received little or no concern for himself as an infant and growing child and therefore had no concern for himself or others as an adult. He could be as frightening and threatening as is possible; he didn't feel fear as he didn't care if he lived. By the time he had come to me, via a sympathetic GP, he had had a lifetime of punishment (in psychiatric hospital as a 16–18 year old), vilification (in the family), dismissal (at school he had been written off as useless), social control (heavy cocktails of prescribed drugs). He had little experience of mattering to anyone and little or no connection with others. It was remarkable, and perhaps speaks of some good internalised early objects (father/elder sister) that he was alive or that he was not in prison for murder.

Initially my work with him was simply about trust. He was wounded, terrified, deeply suspicious and paranoid. He had a long history with the psychiatric services and with several GPs and was not assuming anything when we first met. I had to pass his test. Strangely, although the early months were harrowing and sessions seemed to be on a knife edge as to whether he'd commit or run, I was never frightened *of* him, but I was very frightened *for* him. In therapeutic terms I think back on the work as being quite simple. I simply cared about him. He never liked it when I got too clever – there was no point. We used the time to think about him and we did it together. I failed him at various times by trying too hard to impress or by talking to the psychiatrist without telling him first. Others failed him too during the course of the work – his wife, his GP. And of course he failed himself on many occasions. He went back to carrying a knife after a particularly difficult time with one of the family. He told me that he'd taken it up again and I told him that it was too dangerous for him to carry a knife and that I did not want him to continue to do so. His therapy was in danger if he continued to. He would be jeopardising the good he was letting himself dare to have. He was able to put it away again. It seemed that he heard me saying that he mattered. That was a new experience for R. Much later in the work he gave me the tape. But I think it resonated back to this and many similar moments thereafter.

The song, like most pop songs, has a repetitive cyclical structure with verses and a repeating refrain/chorus. The main phrase that is repeated is 'You needed me'. As an expression of patient to therapist this is quite curious and striking. The rest of the song is made up of lyrics that are on the face of it more understandable in the context and speak of a loving, idealised transference: 'you gave me strength to carry on, you picked me up when I was down . . . so high that I could almost touch the sky', etc. It is on one level a love song. But the oft-repeated refrain 'you needed me ' with its echo later in the song of 'I needed you' is I think where the real meaning lay for R. It is why, when he heard the song, he always thought of me. What I think he was in touch with was that he mattered to me. He was having an experience of being someone who was worthy enough to be the sort of person who is needed by someone else. This was developmental, relational, mutative, transferential, but also real. The act of being someone who someone else wanted to stay alive was transforming for R. He was right – it was love, but of a maternal kind. He had discovered the capacity in himself to evoke love and care from me. The song came out of a very long emotional journey that R had had, as if for the first time. Of course there was with it an adult erotic element, but not exclusively. The choice of song revealed something else other than an ordinary love song. It revealed his need to be needed, to be worthy, to be an effective life, not just a negative life.

Mary asked me why did he choose music to convey his experience of our relationship, as well as why this form of music. I think the music, and in this case also the words of the song, helped R first *recognise* having had something, then *transform* feeling and experience into something which could be expressed and then *shared.* So this is a process from recognition, transformation to relationship.

The second example of music coming into the consulting room is an account by Fiona Aitken.

Fiona Aitken

James, a 30-year-old, white, middle class rock musician, attended private therapy because of relationship breakdown with his partner Joy. The son of two community workers, who were very active in issues of social justice, James grew up in a working class neighbourhood in London. He had always felt 'out of place' and anxious about standing out and being different in the mainly working class school he attended. To alleviate the pain of this as a child he joined in various 'gang' activities which culminated in a court appearance for theft. His parents were mortified. They said little, however, about the incident. James was given a warning but nothing further took place. His parents had had an 'open' marriage and James was accustomed to his parents rowing about various partners involved with the two of them. He felt caught between them, with a role of holding them together. He would manifest this by climbing into bed between them at night.

At secondary school James got involved in music and gained kudos from his talent to write creatively. His involvement in the music industry meant that he got involved in drug usage, including LSD, cannabis, speed and heavy drinking sessions. This had resulted in psychotic episodes, resulting in referral to the local psychotherapy unit. After some short-term intervention, which seemed to stabilise him, he found his way into the private practice arena. I saw him for four years.

James had met Joy, a young black social worker after a concert. Falling madly in love with each other, the pair had set up home rapidly. The relationship was stormy and marked by Joy often walking out in the middle of rows, shouting she was going to find another man, one who could 'really keep his shit together'. The rows occurred after heavy drug/alcohol sessions where one or other of them would feel quite paranoid and accusing.

Over a two-year period, James had an ambivalent attachment to me in the therapy that we had been addressing. This work culminated in him voicing his need for therapy and his anger at me when I failed to be there when he needed me most. This acknowledgement had been accompanied by shame. At the point where music became a major part of our work, I was starting to have romantic fantasies about him. These took the form of sudden unexpected meetings in the local bars; him secretly watching me; me being aware of him but involved with my husband. I would notice a desire to incur jealousy in him. The atmosphere in the therapy room took on the feeling of an affair. I felt as though I was a 'Mrs Robinson' figure (I was 15 years older than James). At this point James was not involved with any women.

James arrived holding out a CD of music performed by his band about to be played on national radio. He featured as the main singer and also wrote the piece.

I didn't play the piece in the room, choosing to listen to it afterwards. It was very arousing, sexy music with a lot of longing expressed in it, with repetitive words describing the wish to make love to the loved one. I enjoyed listening to it and wanted to play it over and over. I noticed I felt secretive about it; I nearly put it on my living room shelves alongside other music, then thought better of it and filed the CD in with my notes. I took the experience of the music to supervision, where my supervisor listened to the music. We both became excited by it. I felt a little like a romantic tryst was being set up with my supervisor as a sort of go-between. We explored this thoroughly.

The next time I saw James, I told him that I had listened to the music. I found it difficult to say anything to him about it because of anxiety about appearing seductive. He looked very coy. I responded by asking him what he was feeling about my having listened to it. He mumbled that he was attracted to me and didn't know if that was 'allowed'. Consumed with shame, James struggled to stay in the room. We processed this over some months and eventually the romantic feelings gave way to another experience.

Six months later, James brought another CD for me to hear. Again, significantly, I didn't play it in the session. The feeling in the music was more varied and at times angry, almost rageful. I experienced tedium this time; it felt like a chore to listen to it and I resented the time it took and found it hard to listen to the music, which I didn't especially like. I had a counter-transferential retaliation, one where I 'forgot' to bring the music back into the room. In a sense it 'festered' in the filing cabinet.

James finally addressed it with me, saying he was angry that I appeared to have neglected it. He shouted, 'have you even heard it!'. I felt caught out and somewhat ashamed as though I had lost something precious of his, a sense of the love affair gone sour.

James elaborated on his anger, telling me it wasn't what the music conveyed this time that was important; more that it was *him* that had produced it. He wanted my admiration that he could produce a whole varied CD. What seemed an issue for him was not what the music conveyed but the CD itself. He wanted me to admire and praise him; being proud of what he could produce. James raged at me about my disregard of his gift to me.

The third account is also by Fiona Aitken.

George was a 50-year-old accountant, who came to see me because he wanted to change careers and become a counsellor. He had applied for a local training and had been asked to attend therapy for his difficulties with a view to re-applying later.

George appeared chaotic, dissociated and had a rather borderline presentation. He had held down his job for ten years and had recently left his partner of five years. George was unable to describe what had led to this parting. He had taken a lot of different drugs in the past but said these 'did my head in' and had stopped over the last few years. Again, all this was somewhat vague. I saw him for two years privately. He had 'serially' seen therapists before, never staying for very long.

George's background was very deprived and filled with abandonment and abuse. Brought up by a young mother of sixteen, he was often found hungry and distressed by neighbours, having been left in his own home alone. He was placed in care from the age of four, where he was sexually abused by one of the male care workers. Finally he was placed with foster parents, and he was again abused by the eighteen-year-old son of his foster parents. George did have contact as a young adult with his mother who was an alcoholic and very self obsessed.

I felt he was much traumatised. This manifestation emerged in a very specific way in the room. As a result I often felt frightened and symbolically 'pinned against the wall' by George's varying manipulations of me. At times I couldn't breathe for feelings of terror and also of shame. When I had opportunities for us to eventually process these experiences, George disclosed that he had worked as a male prostitute when young. This had funded food, accommodation and drugs. George had felt powerful at times because of earning money in this way and had split off the vulnerable experiences of fear and shame that I had held for him. Money and payment of fees to me mirrored some of the dynamics of prostitution, 'paying for love'. George had had a friendship at this time with a salvation army officer. Eventually this man had helped George to 'come off the game'. Following this, George had been supported by his friend to train in accounting and met Ruth, his ex-partner, at work.

George brought music into the room, towards the end of the two-year period and shortly after the processing of the projective identifications from his abuse and period of prostitution. He arrived in the mood of 'Tigger' from *Winnie the Pooh*, bouncing into the room with a guitar in hand. He exclaimed that he had written a song for me and proceeded to play his guitar and sing this song which was all about his feeling of happiness. He looked very young and naïve, quite different from the manoeuvering wiley, pushy man I had been experiencing. I was completely unprepared for this. It was as if I was seeing the boy that would have been there if all the abuse hadn't happened. I was concerned that he had dissociated and split off the experiences we had been working through. Hearing his song, I felt both touched by the sweetness of the words and his manner of bringing it to me. The song also had another mood inherent in it and I was somewhat disquieted. I felt invited into a deal of some kind, a 'grooming'. I experienced being seduced.

In the previous session George had wanted to end his therapy unless I reduced the fee. Confronting this raised ever more powerfully the issue of 'second-hand care', issues of power and paying for love. The 'arrival' of his song seemed incongruent with where we had been together. There was a way in which I felt coerced into listening to it as George didn't contract to bring music and his guitar into the room. I experienced it as both a gift to me *and* tainted with coercion; a breach of boundaries.

I am grateful to Antonia Murphy and Fiona Aitken for describing these three instances of music coming into the consulting room. Music does come into psychotherapy and there is room for different ways of understanding what it might mean for the patient.

Glossary

Affect: Feeling.

Affect regulation: A phrase used to describe the careful attention and attune-ment to the infant's disturbances in feeling and the mother's/carer's appropriate holding and empathic response. Mother's response engages with the infant's intense feelings of rage or relation and enables these to be managed between them. Affect regulation is a dynamic process that is also applicable within the patient/therapist engagement. All aspects of affect regulation are fully covered in Allan Schore's book *Affect Regulation and the Repair of Self* (2003).

Augmentation: A term used in music where the length of the note values in a passage of music is increased from what was sounded earlier. For example, a melody originally consisting of crotchets and quavers (1 beat note values and ½ beat note values) may become a melody of minims and crotchets (2 beat notes values and 1 beat note values).

Communicative musicality: A dynamic motion observed in an infant shortly after birth as it enters into the rhythms and melodies of a conversation. This movement in sound and gesture is with us throughout life when we communi-cate non-verbally and verbally.

Corpus callosum: The fibre tract linking the right and left hemispheres of the brain.

Diminution: A term used in music where the length of the note values in a passage of music is decreased from what was sounded earlier. For example, a melody originally of crotchets and quavers (1 beat note values and ½ beat note values) might become a melody of quavers and semi-quavers (½ beat note values and ¼ beat note values). The whole effect is quickened up.

Dynamic: In energetic motion with a tone or tones in music or in active mental motion with another person or persons.

Dynamic field: *In music*: The 'away from' and 'towards' motion of tones within a passage of music. There will also be a sense of completion or return within the whole piece of music. *In psychotherapy*: The 'away from', 'towards' and 'return' in a new way within the mental dynamics of the relationship between patient and therapist.

Dynamic patterning: The active motion within the form or shape of a group of tones in music and the mirroring of this musical shaping within the mind of the listener or performer. For example, the pattern of feelings in the mind is experienced as corresponding to the flowing pattern in a passage of music.

Enhanced communicative musicality: A phrase used to describe the sound of a passage of music played in the consulting room. Communicative musicality will be already present between patient and therapist in the rhythms and melodies of a conversation both verbally and non-verbally. A passage of music played in the room enhances this communicative musicality further and the music may hold symbolic meanings for the patient. These meanings or metaphors may then enter into the therapeutic conversation.

Feeling: In this book this word is used as a collective term or container for feelings.

Feelings: Particular sensitivities in the mind and body which may alter one's mood. They may also be described as fine-grained nuances of felt experience. One can experience several feelings at the same time.

Fibromyalgia: A musculoskeletal pain with fatigue. The cause of this debilitating illness is still unknown.

Habitus of music: The context of the experience of music along with how it is felt and perceived.

Intrinsic Motive Pulse: A phrase used by Trevarthen to describe the moving and feeling observed in a newborn infant. It is an inborn source in human nature of which psychological science is just beginning to take account.

Music: According to Zuckerkandl, music is motion in the dynamic field of tones. This is a definition which supports the thinking in this book. It is also, according to Langer, a symbol of the shapes and patterns of feeling in our inner mental world. This is also thinking which has informed this book.

Neural pathways: These are the routes of nerve cells in the brain and body.

Pierrot Lunaire (Moonstruck Pierrot): A melodrama for female voices and instruments by A Schoenberg, Opus 21. First performed in 1912.

Psychodynamic psychotherapy: A psychotherapy which is concerned with how early relationships, or lack of them, impacts on the patient's life in the here and now of life. It also influences the relationship with the therapist in the consulting room. When early relationships have been derailed, for whatever reason, the 'good enough' relationship with the therapist assists in the process of therapy and healing and also perhaps transformation for the patient.

Self-in-relationship: A concept rooted in the idea that there is no such thing as a single self, there is only a human self-in-relationship, which can be a positive or negative relationship. There has always been a self-in-relationship from before birth. The idea of single unitary self does arise, however, from the time of birth, but within the self-in-relationship.

Sensate: Bodily sensation and bodily feeling; perceived by the senses.

Stretto: A musical term which means drawn together. This happens, for example, in music that has several voices or parts like a fugue. Stretto is heard when entries of the different voices overlap and are drawn together more closely than when first heard.

Transformational object: A term used by Bollas to describe how an object is experientially identified by the infant as that which will transform his experience. In other words, in a good infant/mother relationship, mother is the first transformational object. Her loving, holding and caring way of being is now understood as leaving brain traces in the adult mind. If this very early experiential process has been derailed, listening to music in adult psychotherapy may again evoke and resonate with these early traces in the patient's brain. This musical process, along with the human presence of the psychotherapist who mirrors the patient's experience of listening to the music, may be a second and familiar transformational experience for the patient.

Index

Abba 14, 61, 124
accessibility and strikingness 62, 63, 167
active music therapy 94–5, 140
Adamenko, Victoria 102
adolescence 84, 85, 111
aesthetic quality 61, 62, 63–4
affect 4, 141, 156, 183
affect regulation 183
affective neuroscience 2, 149, 168
agency 76, 77, 78, 87
Aitken, Fiona 9, 171, 179–82
Almen, Byron 102
alternative cabaret 52
anger 171, 180
Anka, Paul 48
apartheid 20
archetypes 102
Artistic Media and Music Therapy 7, 96, 97
arts
    Bollas 172, 174
    in healthcare 41, 59, 82
    political expression 32
    quality 64, 65
    in therapy 100, 133, 134, 144, 160
attachment
    aural shadow of the object 174
    case study 140, 141, 146–9, 156, 160
    model of mind 168
    origin of aesthetic experience 169
    personal and social identity 85
    self-in-relationship 7, 111
auditory bridge 154
augmentation 8, 183
autonomous splinter psyches 143
autonomy 83–4, 86, 87

Bach, JS
    Baroness Julia Neuberger 36, 38
    case study 124, 133
    everyday and special music 59, 61, 62
    Mercedes Pavlicevic 14
    two-part invention 8
Un Ballo in Maschera (Verdi) 42
Batt, Mike 30, 31, 60, 65
The Beatles
    Baroness Julia Neuberger 38

everyday and special music 60, 61
    Katie Melua 27, 30
    Mercedes Pavlicevic 14, 15
    sociology of experience of music 73
Becker, Judith
    'habitus' of music 6, 93, 94, 166
    model of mind 169
    psychology of experience of music 83, 87
    self-in-relationship 105
    sociology of experience of music 74
Beebe, Beatrice 105, 170
Beethoven, L van 55, 73, 127, 128
Bekkedal, M 2, 112
Belfast (Melua) 31–2, 59
Berg, A 42
Bernatzky, G 103, 106, 112, 113
Bible 48, 49
biocultural evolutionary perspective 74–6
Blacking, J 75
Blood, AJ 113
BMGIM see Bonny Method of Guided Imagery
    in Music
body language 3, 155, 174
Bollas, C 169, 172, 173, 174, 184
Bonde, Lars Ole 7, 96, 98
Bonny Method of Guided Imagery in Music
    (BMGIM) 7, 98, 99, 100, 103
Bonny, Helen 95
Brahms, J
    Baroness Julia Neuberger 35, 36, 38, 44, 57
    everyday and special music 59, 61, 64
    habitus of music 102
    Mercedes Pavlicevic 14, 23
    music and the philosophers 73
brain
    dynamic fields 4
    habitus of music 6
    listening to music 64
    model of mind 168
    music as a universal experience 71
    musical analysis of case study 157, 160, 161
    reflection on case study 139–42, 147–8, 149
    self-in-relationship 7, 110–12, 113, 114
Brandenburg Concertos (Bach) 36, 38
Brit School of Performing Arts 27
Britten, Benjamin 37, 39

186